Carnivore
Diet

I0434671

The #1 Beginners Guide to Weight loss,
Increase Focus, Energy, Fight High Blood
Pressure, Diabetes or Heal Digestive System.

Becky Parker
John Miller

ISBN: 978-0-359-67070-3

Disclaimer Notice:

Please note the information contained within this document is for educational and entertainment purposes only. All effort has been executed to present accurate, up to date, and reliable, complete information. No warranties of any kind are declared or implied. Readers acknowledge that the author is not engaging in the rendering of legal, financial, medical or professional advice. The content within this book has been derived from various sources. Please consult a licensed professional before attempting any techniques outlined in this book.

By reading this document, the reader agrees that under no circumstances is the author responsible for any losses, direct or indirect, which are incurred as a result of the use of information contained within this document, including, but not limited to, — errors, omissions, or inaccuracies.

Table of Contents

Introduction

Congratulations on downloading *Carnivore Diet* and thank you for doing so.

The following chapters will discuss everything that you need to know in order to get started on the carnivore diet. There are a lot of diet plans out there that you can choose to work with. Some are going to be really into cutting out the fats, and others are going to focus more on cutting out the carbs. The ketogenic diet is a very popular diet plan right now and asks the followers to cut out their carbs to almost nothing, and instead consume lots of healthy fats and moderate amounts of protein in order to stay healthy.

With that said, the carnivore diet is a new trend that is taking the world by storm and showing us results that we never imagined in the past. This diet takes the idea of the ketogenic diet and other low-carb diets a step further. It takes us back to our roots, back to focusing on eating foods that our bodies are able to handle, and not to waste time on any other foods that could be harmful to us, or would have taken up more energy than they were worth at the time.

The carnivore diet is one that focuses on eating animal products. You are allowed to eat all of the meat you want, including fish and organs of the animals, butter, and aged cheese. You will need to eliminate the grains, fruits, and vegetables that you consume in order to see the results. This helps you to burn through fat faster, keeps your meals as easy as possible, and can provide you with the health and weight loss benefits you need.

This guidebook is going to take some time to look over the carnivore diet and all of the steps that are needed to become successful in no time. We will look at what the carnivore diet is all about, what foods you are allowed to eat, and which ones you should avoid when you are on this plan, and even some of the amazing health benefits that come with this kind of diet.

From there, we will take it further to look at whether there are any issues or complications that can come with the carnivore diet and how to avoid them, how to add in some exercise to the plan, and even some of the tips that you need to ensure that the carnivore diet is going to provide you with the results that you need.

Sometimes, the hardest part to getting started on a diet plan of any kind, especially one that is as new as the carnivore diet, is figuring out what meals to enjoy. This guidebook is going to end with some delicious breakfasts, lunches, dinners, and sides that you can use to make this diet plan easier, along with a 21-day meal plan so that you are sure you can get on the right foot right out the door with this plan.

When you are ready to see what the carnivore diet is able to do for you, and you are interested in some of the basics that come with it, then make sure that you check out this guidebook and see what is in store for you.

There are plenty of books on this subject on the market, thanks again for choosing this one! Every effort was made to ensure it is full of as much useful information as possible, please enjoy!

What is the Carnivore Diet?

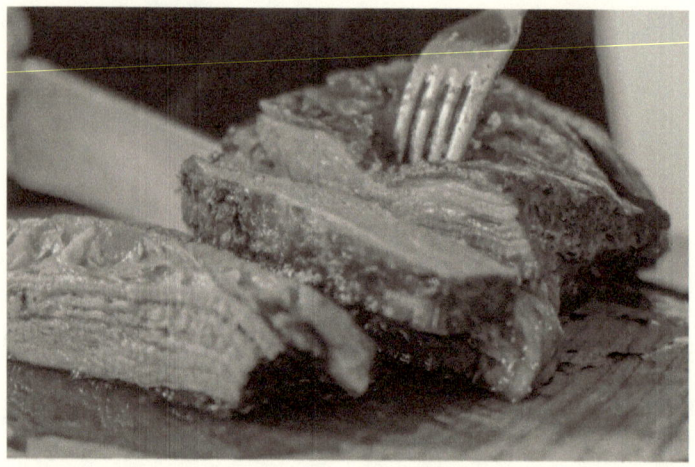

It seems like we are always hearing about a new diet plan that has come out. Each one is going to have different rules and foods that you are allowed to eat and they all seem so different. The Mediterranean diet is all about eating lots of healthy carbs, grains, and vegetables. The vegetarian diet is all about avoiding meat products and enjoying whole grains and produce. Then there is the ketogenic diet that restricts your carbs in favor of lots of healthy fats. And the Paleo diet that wants you to just focus on the foods that your ancestors were able to get ahold of. These are just a few of the different diet plans that are out there, and while each of them promises to provide you with some of the results in weight loss and more that you are looking for, it is time to take a look at the carnivore diet and what it is all about.

The carnivore diet is a new kind of diet that promises to help you lose weight and feel your best in no time. This diet plan asks you to eat no carbs, including no fruits or vegetables. In fact, you will need to focus on just eating meat. But before that inner burger lover starts to jump for joy, it's important to hear some of the details about the diet plan.

The carnivore diet, which is sometimes known as the all meat diet, is going to involve eating almost nothing but meat for every meal *all the time*. This means that you are going to eat a ton of protein, a lot of fat, and almost no carbs at all.

This is going to run against some of the conventional wisdom for nutrition. This means that you will avoid the advice of eating lots of grains, fiber, and vegetables to stay healthy. This advice is a part of many popular diet plans including the vegetarian diet and the vegan diet. Because this diet plan is going to spend so much time focusing on the meats and proteins, with no other options from produce and carbs, you would think that it could cause some issues with weight gain, digestive problems, and high cholesterol levels to name a few of the health problems.

However, this diet plan is proof that conventional wisdom, especially when it comes to health and nutrition, isn't always the right thing to follow. The carnivore diet is going to be based on the idea that our ancestors were able to eat mostly meat, because it wasn't that efficient in terms of energy expenditure to go out and gather a lot of fruits and vegetables. With this idea, it is believed that our bodies have evolved in order to run the best and at its optimum amount, on a diet that revolves around the meats you eat.

According to George Ede MD, there is a historical observation that we can take a look at when comparing the carnivore diet to the vegan diet. This theory is going to help you to really get a good idea on how the carnivore diet is so effective and why you should consider using it for your weight loss goals. The historical observation that helps to support the theory that the carnivore diet from George Ede MD includes:

"To the best of my knowledge, the world has yet to produce a civilization which has eaten a vegan diet from childhood through death, whereas there are numerous examples throughout recorded history of people from a variety of cultural, ethnic, and geographical backgrounds who have lived on mainly-meat diets for decades, lifetimes, generations."

It can sometimes be hard, especially after all of the things that we have heard about how healthy carbs and produce are, to understand how the carnivore diet can be great for your health. Not only does it not cause a lot of harm to the body, but it can actually end up improving your health if you follow it the right way.

Now, this method may not work best for everyone. For example, children should not go on this kind of diet plan because it is important that they get the nutrients that they need from other food sources. Pregnant and breastfeeding women and others who need to monitor their diet with the help of a medical professional will find that it is best to skip out on this diet. For most healthy adults though, the carnivore diet can help them to lose a lot of weight and improve their health while eating foods that are good for them.

What is the Carnivore Diet?

Now that we have taken some time to look at the carnivore diet and what it is all about, it is time to take a closer look at what foods you can eat, the foods that you should avoid, and more.

The ideas of the carnivore diet are pretty simple. This can be a nice thing because many people have trouble going on a diet plan that has so many rules and things attached to it that you can't remember the rules. The simplicity of this diet plan can make it much easier to follow.

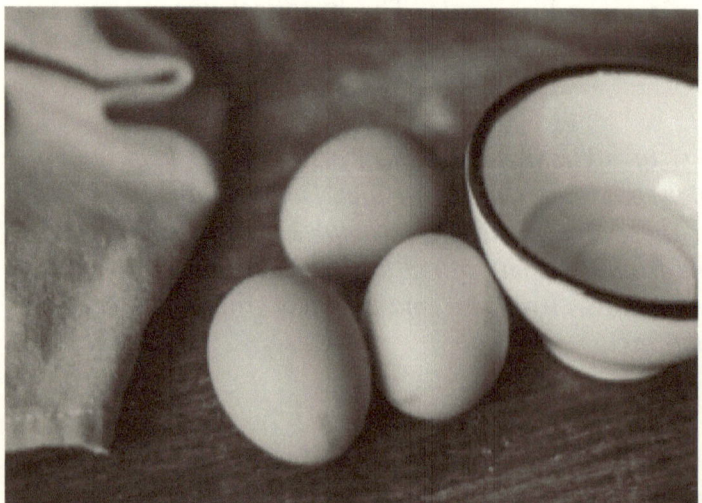

When you are following the carnivore diet, there are four main types of foods that you can consume. Mainly, you are allowed to have meat, cheese, butter, and eggs. You can also eat a few of the zero calorie foods that are available, including spices and coffee. Many people like to work with Bulletproof coffee to give them a little extra energy in the morning, so including something like MCT oil can be allowable in this diet plan as well.

As you can see, when you eat the foods that are above, they are full of protein and lots of fats, but they contain almost no carbs at all. And like some of the other diet plans that are out there, such as the Paleo diet, nuts and vegetables, as well as fruits are need to be avoided because they are going to contain too many carbs in them, and weren't a part of the diet of those we base this diet plan on.

When you are on the carnivore diet, you will need to restrict your carbs. All of your old favorites, from fruits and vegetables to bread, baked goods, and pasta will be cut out. This diet is extremely low-carb. This is such a low number that unless there is a bit of carb in the meat or cheese that you consume, you should not eat any at all. This can be hard to adjust to in the beginning, especially if you are used to having a lot of processed and fast foods in your diet, but it can be really good for your overall health.

The Key Benefits of Going on this Diet Plan

The next thing to focus on when it comes to the carnivore diet is some of the key benefits that come with it. The first benefit that comes with this diet plan is the menu. If you are able to give up your sweet tooth for a diet that is high in meats and some of the other fatty foods that are out there, then this is a good diet plan to work with. You can enjoy a good hamburger and a good steak each day of the week and do well with this kind of diet plan.

Another benefit of using this diet plan is that when you limit your carbs or completely eliminate the number of carbs that you consume, the body is going to enter into a process of ketosis. Ketosis is a type of metabolic process that will result in the body using stored fat as a source of fuel, rather than relying on the carbs that you usually eat. Ketosis has been linked back to a lot of different benefits including helping you gain strength, lose weight, deal with ADHD, and so much more.

The carnivore diet is able to help you to get through the process of ketosis. Also, since it helps to limit the carbs that you consume even more than what you find in traditional diet plans, you will find that you will enter ketosis much faster than with other types of plans. It may take some time to adjust, but going into ketosis can be so amazing for your health and your levels of energy, and it is definitely something that you should aim towards and will achieve with the carnivore diet.

Another benefit of the carnivore diet is that many people find that working in moderation isn't always going to work. They may find that having a little bit of sugar or even a snack is not enough, and you may find that you want to have a lot more. You can try to moderate the amount of sugar that you consume, but the temptation is just too strong. Once you have just a little taste of it, you find that you just give in and have too much.

For these people, the carnivore diet can be a great option because it isn't about moderation when it comes to carbs and sugars. It asks you to completely eliminate these. This can be a great way to adjust to this diet plan and make sure that you are able to lose the weight that you want.

With that said, you need to be aware of a few things here. If you were a heavy into carbs and sugars before the diet plan, the cravings are going to be strong. For the first week or two, you are going to really struggle against the cravings and will have to work hard to fight it. This is because your body likes to have those carbs. They are an easy form of energy that the body can use. But eating these carbs can make you gain weight due to how inefficient the body is to consuming all of the carbs and glucose that you eat, and this results in a lot of extra body fat.

The cravings are going to subside, but you have to be strong enough to fight against them. And this is going to last for a week to two as the body adjusts to the different foods that you eat. Making sure that you stay hydrated and eating enough food to help fill you up and satisfy your energy requirements will ensure that you are going to see results.

The next key benefit that you will be able to receive when you are working with the carnivore diet is that you can lose weight. There are a lot of different success stories about working with the carnivore diet, and it is just going to depend on how much you have to lose. Even those who are in a healthy weight when they started were able to lose six pounds or more in the first few weeks. If you are overweight or obese, it is possible that you could lose even more.

For those who are looking to lose weight and they have tried out different diet plans in the past, the carnivore diet is going to be the answer that you are looking for. It will help you to lose a lot of weight, as long as you are able to eliminate the carbs and sugars in an efficient manner. Once you let go of the cravings and learn how to work with just eating the meats and cheese and butter, you are going to see a big difference in how much weight you can lose, and all of the health benefits that can come with this.

One thing to keep in mind with this diet plan is that it is relatively new. While there have been some great benefits and results that are found with it, it hasn't been around long enough to really get a lot of research done on it. This means that you should use caution with this plan and watch how your body responds. Some people are going to respond well, and others are going to find that it is not quite right for their needs. Learning which one applies to you can take some time and some experimenting.

How to Get Started on the Carnivore Diet

When you are ready to get started on the carnivore diet, there are going to be a few challenges that could come up. There are a few things that you will need to do in order to prepare yourself for getting started on this kind of diet plan and can ensure that you will stay healthy and see results with this diet.

The first thing that you should do when you are considering going on the carnivore diet is to go and visit your doctor. You can discuss a bit about this diet plan and see what their thoughts are on it. The thing that you want to look for here is that you have any health conditions that would make going on this diet plan more difficult or could make it unsafe for you. Your doctor can discuss the diet plan with you and will ensure that you are able to stay healthy when you choose this diet plan.

While you are at the doctor's office, you should also get your blood tested. You will then want to do this blood test two or three months after you get started with your diet plan so that you are able to measure how effective it is. While you can see some weight loss and may notice that you look and feel better, sometimes it is amazing to see the different results that you can get for your health and to see how your blood numbers are doing.

When you get started on your own carnivore diet, start to take note of any of the changes that you notice in your weight, digestion, and energy. You may want to go through and write down how these changes are each day or at least at the end of the week. Everyone is going to be different, even when they go on this diet plan. Writing all of this stuff down can make a big difference in how well you will do with this diet plan and to compare it to how you felt in the beginning.

Next, realize that the first week or two is going to be the hardest. You will need to expect fluctuations in your focus levels, energy, and appetite. You are going to feel amazing with this plan if you are able to stick with it for the long term. But in that first week or so, you may feel hungry, mad, or irritated, and just overall you may not feel good.

This is mostly because you are trying to adjust from using the carbs for energy and going with the fat as your fuel source. This is going to take some time to make some adjustments. If you are able to, pick a week where you are not too busy to get started. See if you are able to work remotely or take some time off so that you can handle your mood swings. See if you can slow down your schedule and see if you are able to sleep in and take it easy. This will make it a bit easier to adjust to this diet plan and can get you on the right track to see the results that you want.

You may need to try and find a little bit of variety as you can. Some people find that they lose their appetite for steak and some of the meat products, but this means you just need to get creative and find the meals that work for you. For example, if you eat a lot of steak in the first week, you may get a bad steak and not like the taste anymore.

This doesn't mean that you should give up on the diet plan altogether. It just means that you need to find some different methods to help you out. You maybe need to add some more cheese and butter into the diet plan or try to eat some more fish and hamburger for a bit. This diet plan does focus a lot on eating steak and more in your eating plan. But if you need a break or changing up a few things, then this is something that you can do.

There are some ways that you can cheat and they can make it a bit easier to work on the diet during the first week. If you do end up cheating, try to not stray too much from the diet plan. For example, while it is not technically allowed on the diet plan, sometimes having a bit of peanut butter is okay. This isn't as bad as going with Twinkies or some of the other options, and it can still give you a lot of the fats and protein that you need as well. Of course, you will need to cut that out as well, but it is a good way to help you adjust if you need a little bit of a cheat while adjusting to the diet plan.

And finally, make sure that you are prepared to some of the appetite swings that you are going to deal with. There are going to be some days where you will hardly eat a thing and not feel hungry at all. And then there are going to be other days where you feel that you are hungry all the time and you just can't get enough to keep you feeling full.

Your appetite is going to start leveling out after the first few weeks. You need to mess around with it and find the right portion sizes that will help you get enough during the day without overeating but will make sure that you don't feel hungry all the time. Until you are able to find this good balance, you should just make sure that you have access to some healthy carnivore-friendly food on all parts of the day. That way, if you aren't hungry, you are set, and if you are hungry, you can grab an extra snack to help you out.

The Difference between the Ketogenic Diet and the Carnivore Diet

While you may look at the carnivore diet and think that it sounds pretty similar to the ketogenic diet, there are actually several differences that can come up. The first difference is that with the ketogenic diet, you need to keep your carbs down, but the carbs that you do eat should come from as many green vegetables as you can. With the ketogenic diet, there is still a belief that produce is good for you, and since the green vegetables can provide you with the nutrients that you need while still being low in the carb department, you will still be encouraged to have some of these.

On the other hand, the carnivore diet doesn't allow for any vegetables at all. It isn't a matter of staying within a certain carb content on the carnivore diet. It is about avoiding carbs *completely*. You should not consume any fruits or vegetables while you are on this kind of diet plan, which is the first reason that it is different from the ketogenic diet.

The second difference is the macronutrient composition of the two diets. With the ketogenic diet, your macronutrient ratio is going to be comprised of about 75 percent fat, 5 percent carbs, and 20 percent protein based on how many calories you are allowed to have each day. However, with the carnivore diet, there isn't really going to be a ratio for the macronutrients. Instead, the follower is asked to just focus their attention on eating fatty meats and then the rest will just fall into place.

Now, if you went through and actually took a look at the macronutrients of what you were eating on a typical carnivore diet, you would find that it comes out to a higher protein allocation and less fat than what is found on the ketogenic diet. But the carb intake would also be a lot lower as well.

With the ketogenic diet, you are asked to be careful with the amount of protein that you consume. You can enjoy some and it is encouraged, but you can also get healthy fats from other sources such as from dairy products and oils. On the carnivore diet, you are asked to only have cheese as a dairy product and butter as your oil, and the rest should come from healthy sources of protein. This is why the ratios of protein and fats may be a bit different.

And the third difference that you may notice when you go on the carnivore diet compared to the ketogenic diet is the use of dairy products. The ketogenic diet is usually going to restrict the amount of dairy products, and often asks you to not consume any because there are some carbs inside. However, since milk and dairy are animal products, the carnivore diet will allow them.

With this said, the carnivore diet will usually ask you to stick with mainly aged cheese rather than milk or other options. You can have them on occasion, but for the most part, butter, eggs, fatty meats, and some aged cheese will be what you enjoy the most on the carnivore diet.

Common Questions about the Carnivore Diet

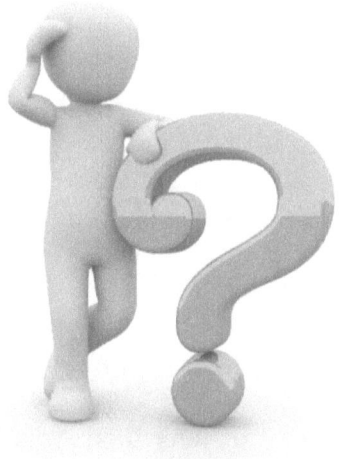

It is normal to have a lot of questions when it comes to following the carnivore diet. It is quite a bit different than what we are used to finding in a lot of the other diet plans out there. And because of this, you will likely have a lot of questions to go with it. Some of the most important questions that can come when someone is just getting started with the carnivore diet include:

Do I really need to eliminate all vegetables?

We have been told that vegetables and fruits are so important for our overall health. We have been told about this our whole lives. But some research has found that vegetables aren't really as important as we have been told for our lives. They do come with a ton of good nutrients and vitamins, but there are other sources of these same minerals, and the produce that you eat may not be the best source.

According to High Steaks, these fruits and vegetables may come with lots of healthy minerals, but they can also come with a lot of anti-nutrients at the same time. These anti-nutrients tend to bind to the same receptors and they can reduce how well the minerals that are good can be taken into the body. Some of the nutrients in the produce will be destroyed by the cooking process, and some are utilized in such a way that we won't be able to absorb and use them without the presence of certain fats in the first place.

Will I experience some digestive problems on the carnivore diet?

Some people worry that when they get started on the carnivore diet, they are going to run into some issues when it comes to not eating any vegetables or anything that contains fiber. There are some people who do notice small disturbances in their digestion. But many found that these disturbances actually went away when they decided to go on the carnivore diet. For most people though, these digestive problems aren't going to show up, even though you are eating fewer products that contain fiber.

Will I need to take a fiber supplement while on this diet plan?

If you are not taking in a lot of junk food, which is something that will naturally happen on the carnivore diet, then you won't need to take in a ton of fiber. An analogy that goes with this is this: Tylenol might be helpful to someone experiencing neck pain, but might not be helpful to someone who is not experiencing neck pain, or it could even cause some side effects that are negative to those who don't need it.

Isn't it bad for you to eat a lot of red meat?

Like many things in nutrition, as well as in your life, you have to consider some of the other variables that are in play when some people are told they shouldn't eat red meat. If you eat a lot of sugar, don't get out and exercise on a regular basis, and you eat red meat, then it is likely that you won't be that healthy of a person. But, if you eat a lot of red meat, avoid sugar, exercise, and eat other foods that are healthy, then the red meat is not going to be harmful.

Should I worry about my cholesterol levels?

There's a bit of a debate about whether meat and fat are going to cause your cholesterol levels to go up. However, there are a lot of variables that come into play when you are talking about cholesterol and for everything that is in our bodies for that matter. If you are eating a lot of sugar and a lot of fat at the same time, this is going to be a different scenario compared to eating a lot of fat without any sugar.

In fact, there are a lot of studies out there that show how fat isn't the main culprit to the health conditions that we often suffer from. Instead, it is the sugar that is causing these issues. Correlation, of course, isn't going to mean causation. Exercise is another important thing to consider here. Getting your body up and moving, rather than always staying inside and doing no activity can even affect your cholesterol levels as well.

There are a lot of questions that come up when you hear about the carnivore diet. It is a very healthy diet, one that asks you to follow what is natural for the body by eating mostly meat, along with healthy butter and cheeses, and reduce your carbs to pretty much nothing. While it does go against a lot of the different things that we know when we talk about traditional dieting advice, it is going to make some big changes in how your health is doing.

What Foods Can I Eat on the Carnivore Diet?

Now that we know a bit more about the carnivore diet plan, it is time to take a closer look at some of the foods that you are allowed to eat when you are on this diet plan. This one can be difficult to work with sometimes because there are so many restrictions. But it is also seen as an easy option to go with because you only have to remember about four foods that you are allowed to eat. For those who want quick results without a ton of limitations and rules that go with it, then the carnivore diet is the right option for you. Let's take a look at some of the foods that you are allowed to eat, and some of the foods that you should avoid when you go on the carnivore diet.

The Foods You Can Eat

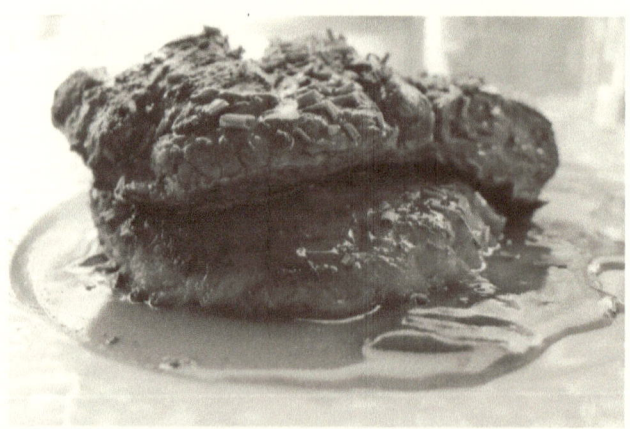

The food group that you need to focus on the most when you go on the carnivore diet is the fatty meats that you consume. In fact, the majority of your calories are going to come from fatty meats. There are a lot of options that come with this, and since it provides you with the healthy fats and protein that you need to still have plenty of energy each day, there is nothing wrong with eating enough until you are full and satisfied.

There are a lot of different options of meats that you are allowed to consume when you are on this kind of diet plan. Some of the beef cuts that you should focus on (and beef is the meat source that is the most highly recommended when you are on this diet plan), includes:

1. Organs from the animals. This is not required but can help mix things up if you would like.
2. Ground beef
3. Roasts. This includes options like brisket, chick, and prime rib.
4. Steaks. You can enjoy almost any kind of steak that you would like including chuck eye, strip, sirloin, and ribeye.

A note about the organ meats: There are some of those on this diet plan who believe that you need to eat the organ meats in order to get all of the nutrition that is needed on this diet plan. However, this isn't a requirement of the diet plan. While there are a lot of great benefits of consuming these meats and you can get many extra nutrients plus switch up and add some variety to your diet plan, eating organ meat is not a requirement if you don't feel consuming it on this diet plan.

Of course, you don't have to limit yourself to just consuming beef as your own meat source on this diet plan. You are also allowed to consume options like lamb, pork, poultry, and fish.

There are a few options when you are picking out the beverages that you want to consume on this diet plan. You will be limited a bit because things like sodas and alcohol are not allowed at all. These are going to contain some extra carbs and sugars that are not good for you, especially on this diet plan, so you need to eliminate them.

The primary source of hydration that you should enjoy on the carnivore diet is water. You are allowed to have it plane or choose to go for mineral water or carbonated water. Other options include bone broth, tea, and coffee.

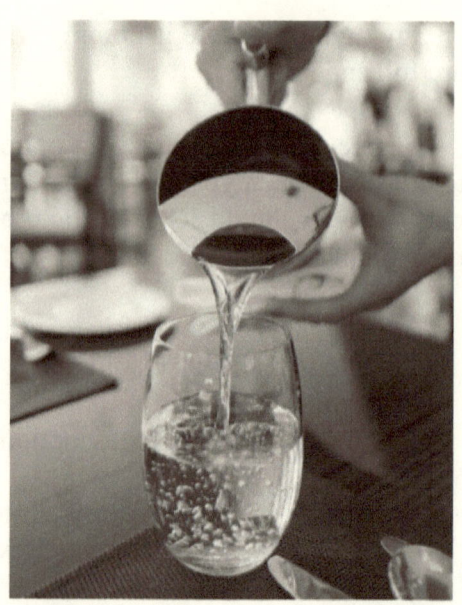

In addition to getting to enjoy a lot of great sources of fatty meats, you can enjoy a few other options as well. This is going to include hard cheeses, heavy whipping cream, butter, and eggs. You can implement these into your diet plan as much as you would like, along with some healthy spices as much as you would like. With some tasty combinations of these, you are going to be able to enjoy many varieties and meals while on this diet plan.

The Foods That You Should Avoid

The list of foods that you need to avoid when you are on the carnivore diet is going to be pretty long. You will find that there are many different types of foods that you need to be careful about when you are on this diet plan because they are going to contain too many carbs, or they just don't work with what our ancestors may have eaten in the past. And, according to the rules of this diet plan, this means that your body is not optimized for dealing with these other foods, even though they are commonly found in the American diet.

The first group of food that you need to keep out of your diet plan will be the carbs. Many people like to have carbs with their meals. They like to
have the cereals, the grains, bread, and pasta for their meals. According to traditional nutritional advice, the whole grains are seen as a good thing and provides the body with the healthy fiber and B-vitamins that are needed.

Since these whole grains are going to be too full of carbs and there are more efficient sources of these nutrients compared to the whole grains, it is time to reduce them on the carnivore diet. In fact, it is recommended that you avoid these as much as possible because they will ruin you being in the process of ketosis. You need to find other options that are seen as better for the carnivore diet, and learn how to say goodbye to some of the whole grains that you enjoyed in the past.

You also need to avoid the fruits and vegetables that you enjoyed in the past. There are a lot of things that you can enjoy about having fresh produce, but these need to be eliminated when you are on this diet plan. They have healthy nutrients that can be good for your body, but they also have a lot of anti-nutrients that can cause other problems in the body.

There is also the added issue of the body not being able to consume or absorb some of the nutrients that are in the produce you consume, without having some fat there to help with the absorption. This means that you could eat all of the fruits and vegetables that you want, and if you don't take in enough of the healthy fats that you need, then you are just going to waste all of those good nutrients.

When you are on the carnivore diet, you need to reduce and eliminate the amount of fresh produce that you are consuming on a regular basis. This can be hard, especially if you got familiar with eating lots of healthy nutrients from them in the past. But since there are better ways to get the healthy nutrients that are found in produce (mainly from the healthy meats that you should consume above), you need to get them out of your diet plan as soon as possible.

You also need to be careful about all of the baked goods and processed foods that you are used to consuming on the traditional American diet. If you eat a lot of carbs and sugars and you like to have baked goods on a regular basis, then this is one that will be hard to work with. You will find that you may have to deal with some sugar cravings and sugar withdrawals, which can make giving these things up almost impossible.

But if you really want to see the results that are promised with this diet plan, there are lots of healthy and tasty foods that you can consume instead, so you should focus on those instead of letting yourself miss the foods that are listed above.

Getting used to the carnivore diet is going to take some time, and it can sometimes become difficult for someone to get used to it. The unhealthier the foods you enjoyed on your diet plan when you first got started on the carnivore diet, the harder those first few weeks are going to be.

The good news is that once you get adjusted to this new way of eating, once you learn how to get over those sugar cravings, once you see the new energy you can enjoy from the process of ketosis, and once you learn that there really are a lot of options when you get on this diet plan to help provide you with some variety and lots of good tastes, you will soon see the benefits not just on your weight, but in your overall health as well.

What about the beverages?

When it comes to working with the carnivore diet, you have to be careful about the types of beverages that you are allowed to consume. For the most part, you will need to make sure that you are keeping mostly water as your primary source of hydration. When you switch over to eating a diet that is mostly animal products, you are going to feel thirstier than you did in the past. It is important that you are keeping some water by you at all times and to drink plenty so you don't become dehydrated.

You are allowed to enjoy plain water, mineral water, and carbonated water. However, you can't go through and add a lot of things to the water. This means no flavorings, and no fruits and vegetables added to make it taste better. Just stay with plain water to make sure that you are getting the hydration that you need, without all the added stuff.

Next, you are also allowed to consume some green tea (in some versions of the carnivore diet, although there are some that cut this out), some coffee (as long as it doesn't have any additives to it like creamer and sugar), and bone broths. There are some methods that are going to allow milk since this is an animal product, but others will cut it out because it is going to have too many carbs inside.

There are a number of beverages that you will need to cut out from your diet to make sure that you see success. You will need to cut out all forms of alcohol. These are made out of fruits and grains in most cases, and neither of these is allowed on the carnivore diet. You will also need to take out fruit juices, most milk, and all kinds of sodas.

Can we have spices?

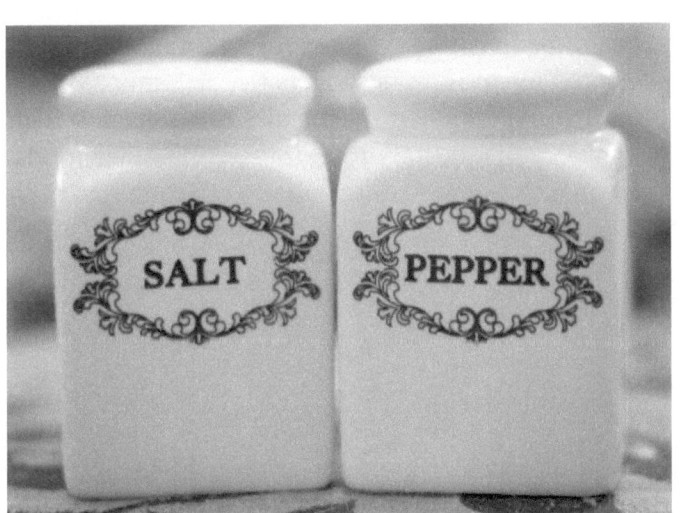

There are some spices that you are allowed to have on this diet plan. Most of the spices are allowed for the carnivore diet, and they can add in some more flavoring to the mix and can change up some of the meals that you decide to have with the carnivore diet. For the most part though, salt and pepper are the two most widely used spices on this kind of diet plan, and many of the recipes that you choose to work with are going to include those two spices inside of them.

With that said, you should be careful about the amount of salt that you use on some of your meals. If you are already dealing with high blood pressure, then limiting the amount of salt that you consume can be a good thing. And even if you aren't currently worrying about high blood pressure because it hasn't been an issue for you in the past, you should still try to limit the salt intake to ensure that you don't have to worry about high blood pressure.

There are a lot of other types of spices that you should consider as well. If you want to avoid the salt so that you can protect your high blood pressure, you will be able to choose some of those spices to help add some more flavor on your meals, without the problems from the salt.

When it comes to using other condiments, you will need to eliminate those completely. You can work with bone broth and that sometimes adds a bit of flavoring and can be a kind of sauce for you. But condiments are not an animal product, they are high in sugars and carbs, and there isn't really anything in them that is healthy, so you need to keep them out of the carnivore diet plan.

Making sure that you eat the right types of foods is so important to help you get the health benefits that you are looking for. The list of foods that you are allowed to eat is any products that are animal made and nothing else. When you are able to make sure that you stick with these kinds of foods and you learn how to eliminate the other foods, you are going to see some amazing results with your health and with some weight loss.

What are the Health Benefits of the Carnivore Diet?

If you were trying to design a new diet plan, one that was for those who didn't need to eat carbs and who didn't like to eat a lot of fruits and vegetables, the carnivore diet would be the answer that you are looking for. This diet plan is going to focus primarily on dealing with just fatty sources of meat for your fuel. There are a few other options that you can make when it comes to going on this diet plan, but for the most part, you will need to focus your dietary efforts on healthy sources of meat, eggs, some dairy, and spices.

This diet may be quite a bit different than we are used to seeing on the traditional diets out there, and it may fly in the face of some of the conventional wisdom that we see when working on our health and fitness. But it is so effective and can help us to get in the best health of our lives. Some of the different health benefits that you will be able to see when you choose to switch out the traditional American diet with the carnivore diet include:

Lose weight

The number one reason that a lot of people choose to go on the carnivore diet is because they are
looking to lose weight. When you go on an all-meat diet, one of the first reactions that you may have about it is that these foods are going to make you fat. But it has been shown that this is highly unlikely. Just like with being on the ketogenic diet, when you eliminate the carbs that you eat, you will be able to make sure that

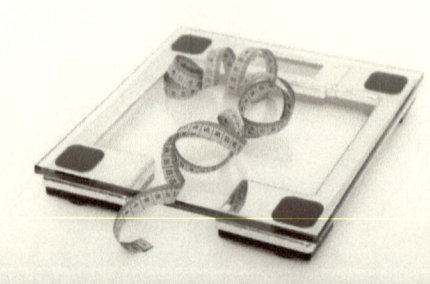

your blood sugar levels are kept to a low amount at all times. You won't have to deal with any of the spikes of the insulin, so there is no reason for the body to store any of the calories that you consume as body fat. In addition, the limitations on what you are allowed to eat with this diet plan can make it really hard to take in too many calories without having to work really hard to make it happen.

If you are someone who will absent-mindedly eat on snack foods, pretzels, and nuts, which mean that you will take in hundreds of extra calories without noticing, then the carnivore diet is going to help you to keep things in check. You have to actually prepare the foods that you are going to eat, because there isn't much room for snack foods, at least not ones that are easy to make. When you think about all of the extra work that you have to put in to just make the meal, you learn how to only eat when you are really hungry.

It may be easy to throw down the snack foods without thinking about it, but it is never by accident that you cook up a steak or a hamburger. This means that you have to take some effort in order to see the results that you want here. You will learn to eat only when you need to, and you can learn how to just take in the number of calories that are needed to sustain you, without overeating. You will, most importantly, learn the difference between mindless eating and physiological hunger.

Many of those who choose to go on the carnivore diet will find that they are able to lose a lot of weight. They are learning how to only eat the foods that they need while avoiding lots of high calorie and processed foods that they were eating before. When these come together, you are bound to see some great weight loss with this plan.

Help your heart get healthier

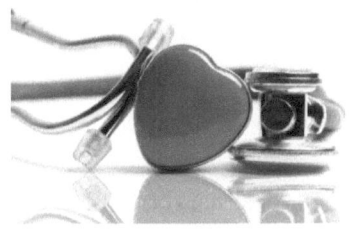

Another great benefit that you are able to get when you are working with the carnivore diet is that it can help to protect the heart. According to the Mayo Clinic, the ratio of your cholesterol is going to be a better risk predictor than the total cholesterol or the LDL. To find this, you would need to go in and divide the total cholesterol number that you had by the HDL score. This is going to be different based on the numbers that you get.

Another thing to consider about your cholesterol is that even though the higher LDL numbers are often seen by doctors as risky, the type of LDL particles that are going through your veins and arteries will be more important than that number. If the particles are small and denser, then they are going to be seen as more dangerous compared to if they are bigger and fluffier. This is why there can be two individuals with the same value of LDL, but their risks are going to be different.

According to the Cooper Institute, the best way to determine the type of particles of LDL that you have is to find your ratio of triglycerides to the HDL cholesterol. The lower this ratio is, the less risk you are dealing with.

For those who went on the carnivore diet, these ratios all went down. Even though there is a lot of controversies that can come from following this diet plan, and many are worried that it is going to be an unhealthy one to choose, especially when it comes to your cholesterol levels, it has actually proven to be different. Being on the carnivore diet can actually reduce the right numbers and increase the right numbers along the way. This can help you to see some great benefits, without having to give up the diet plan.

Some of the other ways that you can see benefits when working with this diet plan and how it can work to keep your heart strong include reducing your blood pressure, opening up the arteries a bit to pump blood through better, and reducing your risk of diabetes. When all of these come together, it can show you just how great your heart health can be and ensures that your longevity is going to increase.

Can help fight off diabetes

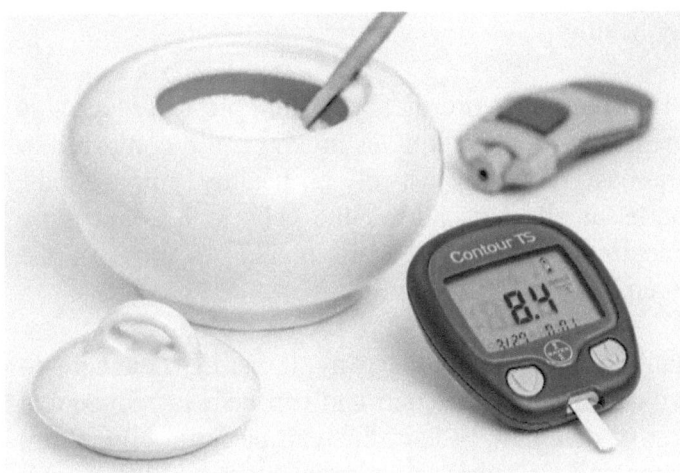

Diabetes is quickly starting to become an epidemic in many different individuals. It is a hard one to deal with, and it can be hard to live a life that is healthy enough to keep you from developing more complications from this condition. The good news is that the carnivore diet is able to help prevent and reduce your risk when it comes to diabetes.

Diabetes is a condition that occurs when we take in too much glucose. This glucose can come from too much sugar and too many carbs since both are going to be converted into glucose in the body. The cells like to use glucose as a form of energy, but when we take in too much, the cells end up not needing as much but the glucose is still there.

Now, when glucose is brought into the body, the liver is going to produce some insulin in order to alert the cells that there is some extra energy available and to let it in. If you eat a healthy diet, then this process is going to work well. But when you take in too much glucose, the cells can become resistant to the insulin. This means that the cells need to have more insulin before they recognize it is there. The liver will continue to produce more, and the cells will become more and more sensitized in the process.

Over time, the cells are barely going to recognize the insulin at all. There will be plenty of glucose there and the cells will need the glucose, but because the cells are so sensitized to the insulin, the glucose will never be absorbed. This result in a high blood sugar level, which can start to damage the body and the individual is going to wear down and feel tired because it is not receiving the nutrients that it needs to stay healthy.

When you go on the carnivore diet, you are able to reduce this issue. First, you are going to stop eating as much insulin compared to what you did in the past. You will just rely on healthy animal foods, rather than any carbs at all. This allows the cells to become more sensitive to the insulin and they will start to take up more of the glucose that had been ignored in the past.

If this diet plan is used in the proper way, it can help the cells to gain their sensitivity to the insulin again and can help to reduce and eliminate the issues of diabetes. In fact, this can be more efficient at dealing with diabetes and the other issue in the body without having to take a lot of bad medications or having to constantly worry about your high blood sugars any longer.

Fewer problems with inflammation

Inflammation is going to be a big issue for many individuals. In fact, it is one of the underlying reasons that we are dealing with a lot of the health conditions that are so prevalent today. Finding ways to reduce the amount of inflammation that we are dealing with on a regular basis can make such a big difference in our overall health.

According to some of those who choose to go on a vegan diet, eating lots of foods that are considered animal foods and are high in fat are going to promote inflammation. They often take it so far as to say that the inflammation that comes from the animal foods that you eat is as high as that inflammation you will get while smoking cigarettes.

The truth is that these kinds of foods can actually go a long way at lowering the amount of inflammation that is in the body. In one 2013 study that was shown in the Journal Metabolism, subjects were compared. The participants were split up into two groups, those who ate high-fat and low-carb diet, and then those who ate high-carb and low-fat diet. The calories were restricted for both of the groups, but the high fat eaters ended up having lower markers of inflammation after 12 weeks of this program.

Because of the results of this study, the researchers were able to conclude that eating more fats and fewer carbs could be more beneficial to the health of the heart and for reducing inflammation throughout the body.

Why does this happen? The liver is going to produce what is known as CRP or C-reactive proteins when there is inflammation in the body. It is possible to measure the amounts of CRP in the blood and use this number to figure out how much inflammation is going on in the system. A level that is at 10mg/L or less is pretty normal, and if you can stay at 1mg/L or less, that is really good.

When the blood levels of the participants in the high-fat group were tested, it was found that they ended up with a CRP score that was really low. Many of them averaged at 0.34. This is an amazingly low number and shows that by going on a low-carb diet and eating lots of healthy fats instead could be the key that we need to reduce how much inflammation we are dealing with, and can ensure that we are able to get the health results, such as relief from high blood pressure, diabetes, cholesterol, and more, that we are looking for.

Higher levels of testosterone

Some of those who have gone on the carnivore diet will discuss how they are going to have higher levels of testosterone. Diets that are high in healthy fats have been shown to help boost the levels of testosterone in any individuals. In fact, there is a study that was done in the American Journal of Clinical Nutrition that found how men who were able to follow a low-fiber and high-fat diet for at least ten weeks, would end up with a total testosterone levels that were 13 percent higher, compared to those subjects who ate low fat and low fiber.

If you have struggled with fertility or with your levels of testosterone, then it may be worth your time to learn more about this diet plan and figure out how you can implement it into your own life.

There are so many things to love about this diet plan, and the fact that it can increase the testosterone levels of men, especially for those who have struggled with it for a long time, is truly amazing.

If you have been dealing with low levels of testosterone and having trouble with getting gains at the gym or your sex life has gone down a bit, then having a boost to your testosterone could be beneficial. Having some increase in the testosterone could be something that you need to spend a bunch of money with getting medication that could be high in bad side effects, or you can choose to start eating more meat and go on the carnivore diet to see the results that you want.

Increases your HDL cholesterol levels

There are two main types of cholesterol. There is the LDL cholesterol, which is the one that is responsible for carrying cholesterol from your liver out to the rest of the body. This is considered the bad type of cholesterol, the one that most people want to avoid as much as possible. The lower you can keep this number, the healthier you will be.

On the other hand, the HDL cholesterol that we are talking about here is the good one, the kind that will carry cholesterol away from the body and puts it in the liver. The liver is then able to reuse or get rid of the cholesterol so it no longer causes any harm to the body.

When you are on the carnivore diet, your levels of triglycerides are going to decrease while your levels of HDL are going to increase. The triglyceride HDL ratio is often a strong indicator of heart disease. The higher this ratio is, the greater your risk of heart disease. But since the carnivore diet is able to help reduce this ratio, it can actually help to benefit your body in so many ways.

Appetite control

One thing that you will be amazed about when you start on the carnivore diet is that you won't feel as hungry as you did before.

Also, you won't end up with a lot of random cravings for things that are bad when you are on this diet. The first week or so is hard while the body adjusts and learns how to handle not getting as much food as before. But after that time, you will be able to control your appetite and not want to reach for the bad stuff as often.

Because of this appetite control, many of those who start on a carnivore diet will also be able to do a form of intermittent fasting, where they are going to limit their eating window and extend their time without eating. This is easier to do on the carnivore diet than some others because your stomach won't rumble all the time and try to convince you to reach for some of the tasty, but unhealthy snacks that you love.

For those who are constantly worried about being hungry and who dislike going on a diet plan because they worry about how hungry they are going to feel, the carnivore diet can be the right option for you. The meals that you get to eat on this diet plan can be filling and will ensure that you get full faster. This helps you to feel better while dieting and can encourage more weight loss in less time.

Fewer digestive problems

One of the main issues that people worry about when they get started with the carnivore diet is whether they are going to be able to provide their bodies with the amount of fiber that is needed. We have been told constantly that we need to eat a lot of fiber. We have seen advertisements for Metamucil and bran muffins that talk about we need to make sure that you consume enough fiber to help our digestion work the proper way. However, when you are on the carnivore diet, fiber is often going to be seen as more trouble than it is worth. And there may be some science out there to prove this as true.

According to a study that was done in 2012 in the World Journal of Gastroenterology, the researchers took the time to investigate the effects of reducing the amount of fiber to people with chronic constipation. Of course, this is against everything that we have been told in the past that is healthy, and it is against what many doctors would recommend.

During this study, the subjects were told to take in minimal amounts to no fiber for the two-week period. They were then, after that time passed, able to increase their fiber intake to a level that they were the most comfortable with. And some were allowed to follow a high fiber diet if they decided that was the best option for them.

What is amazing is that many of the participants of this study found that they were feeling better when they went back to the plan that had zero fiber because it made them feel the best. And this was over a six-month period. Those who were put on the high fiber diet reported that there weren't any changes to their condition. But for those who at either no, or at least smaller amounts of fiber, found that there was a bit improvement in the symptoms that they felt, including symptoms like straining, bloating, and reduced gas. In addition, the ones who were able to decrease their fiber to nothing, or close to nothing, saw that there was an increased level of frequency in how many bowel movements they had each day.

So, how is this possible? How is it possible that eating lower amounts, and sometimes even not eating fiber at all, could help to improve digestive problems when the fiber is supposed to be the thing that makes the digestive system works the best.

The reason that fiber filled eating ends up being problematic for a lot of people and for their stomachs still isn't clear. But many dieters on the carnivore diet are going to blame certain compounds that are found in the plant foods as the main source of these digestive issues. In a book by Steven R. Gundry M.D., The Plant Paradox, it is argued that the natural defense mechanisms that come in plants are going to cause bloating, gas, and some of the other digestive distresses that can make them a bad dietary choice for most humans.

There are a lot of plants that need to be avoided in order to make sure that the body is not going to react in a negative manner to the fiber and other nutrients inside. You should watch out for seeds, nuts, grains, beans, greens, and fruits because these can contribute to inflammation throughout the body as well as to some auto-immune disorders.

While this is going to be an opinion that is still seen as highly controversial, it could really explain why so many carnivore dieters claim that they feel so much better when they are on this diet plan compared to how they felt when they did eat plants. Most of us have been told for a long time that fiber is so important and that we need to consume it in order to stay healthy. But maybe this isn't true. The carnivore diet that we have been discussing is going to challenge a lot of what we think we know about this topic.

Lower blood pressure

If you have ever dealt with issues of blood pressure in your life, then you know how important it is to try to improve those numbers and keep yourself as healthy as possible. The longer that the blood pressure is high and the higher the numbers, the worse it can be not only for your heart but also for your overall health.

High blood pressure is one of the earliest signs of future problems with 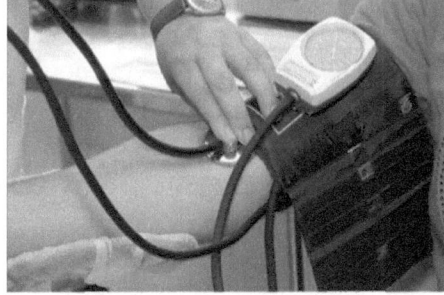 your heart. The carnivore diet does a great job at helping you to lower your high blood pressure, without needing medications to help. In fact, if you are able to actively follow the ketogenic diet, then it will be easy to lower your blood pressure and even stop taking some of your blood pressure medication.

There are a lot of medications out there that you can go on to help lower your blood pressure levels. Some of these are going to work, but most of them will not provide you with the benefits that you are looking for. And even the ones that work can have a lot of negative side effects that can be worse than the high blood pressure and can make a lot of people who are on them even sicker than they were to start with.

One of the best things that you can do is work on your diet to help lower the amount of high blood pressure that you are dealing with. And no diet out there is more effective at helping lower these numbers than the carnivore diet. This diet plan helps you to reduce the amount of salt that you consume, helps you to reduce the amount of processed and fast foods that you eat, and encourages you to eat healthier. When all of these factors come together and when you start to add in some good exercise to the mix as well, you are going to see some amazing results with your health, including your high blood pressure.

More energy

Your body is only able to store so much glycogen at a time. Because of this, you will need to refuel all the time in order to help keep up some of your energy levels. However, most people have plenty of fat for the body to work on, and since the body is efficient at storing more fat than glycogen, it is never going to run out when it is in ketosis.

Imagine how much extra energy you could enjoy on a regular basis. Many people are worried that fat is bad for them and that they need to avoid it at all costs. But in reality, as long as you choose healthy fats that are good for you, you will actually end up with more energy in the long run.

All of us would like to have more energy on a regular basis. We are constantly running around trying to get enough things done. Between work, cleaning the house, getting the kids from school, meeting up for appointments, seeing friends and family, and getting everything done on a regular basis, it is no wonder that we have a lot of trouble keeping our energy levels high and feeling like we can keep up with the day.

Most people are going to rely on lots of coffee and energy drinks to help them make it through the day. While these can work for a bit, they often wear out way before we would like, and it can lead to a big crash that leaves us feeling worse than we did before. These are not the best to use to help us gain and maintain the energy that we need.

The carnivore diet can help us get the right energy, at the right time, without all of those harsh crashes. In the first week or so, you may feel a bit worn out as the body makes some changes and tries to get used to the new diet plan. But once the adjustments start to show up, you will be amazed at the amount of natural energy you will have to help you get through the day.

Increased mental clarity

Just like you can see when you are going on the ketogenic diet, those who choose to go on the carnivore diet are going to notice that their focus and mental clarity are able to increase almost right away. Now, you may notice that when you first get started on this diet plan, there is going to be a period of time when your body has to make some adjustments. If you were a heavy carb eater in the beginning before you switched over to this diet plan, then this adjustment period is going to be worse. During this time, you may have brain fog, be moody, and feel lethargic all at the same time.

In addition, there are some people who develop other negative side effects at the same time as they make these adjustments along the way. You may find that you have some trouble sleeping and you could develop some bad breath, which is an early sign that the body is making some ketones and you are entering the process of ketosis. Once this happens, your energy levels are going to start coming back.

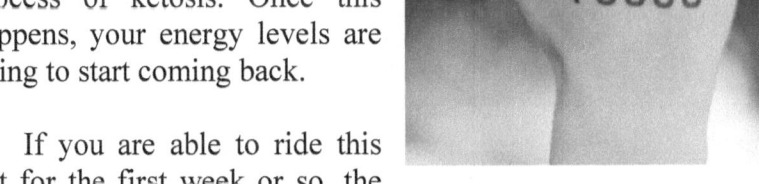

If you are able to ride this out for the first week or so, the side effects are going to fade. You will notice that after this time, your mind is going to feel sharper, and you may even notice more mental clarity and more energy than what you found if you tried working with the standard ketogenic diet.

It is a simpler form of dieting

There is one thing that you can find about the carnivore diet that no one is really able to argue with and it is not really that complicated at all. When you feel hungry, you eat animal foods and that is the end of it. If you are someone who doesn't like the idea of going on a diet plan that is endlessly complicated, someone who gets confused worrying about calories or all of the macros that you need to keep track of, who doesn't want to learn about gluten-free and what that entails, and you don't want to waste your life weighing portions out on a food scale, then this diet plan is the right one. It makes dieting simple because there are very few things to remember.

When you are on this diet plan, you don't have to worry about measuring anything out. You just eat when you are hungry and learn to stop eating when you are no longer hungry. You can certainly go through and measure out the portions and see how big they are if you are curious, but if you learn how to listen to your body and the cues that it can send out, you will find that it is an easy diet plan to follow because you don't have to remember a lot of rules.

You will find that, despite how it sounds, you won't end up eating too much on this diet plan. The foods that you are allowed to have on this diet plan will be low in carbs and high in fats. These fats are very good at filling you up, and this can mean that you take in fewer calories overall. While you are going to feel very full and satisfied on this diet plan, you will find that you aren't taking in nearly as many calories as you did in the past, and this is what helps you to lose weight in the process.

As you can see, there are a lot of health benefits when it comes to following the carnivore diet. You will find that it is quite a bit different than what you may have been used to in the past. But once you get familiar with the carnivore diet plan and you learn the rules about what you can and can't eat, it is actually a simple plan. You don't have to remember a ton of rules, and you get the benefit of seeing your health improve in no time at all.

Are there Any Complications with this Diet Plan?

Since the carnivore diet is similar to the ketogenic diet and we have already seen how meat isn't the only thing that you can blame for heart disease, it is safe to assume that this kind of diet plan is going to be safe for most people to enjoy, at least over the short term.

However, there are a lot of myths out there about eating an all meat diet, and how it can be bad for your overall health. The good news is that most of these are just myths, and there is no scientific proof behind any of it. For example, let's take a look at the idea that meat can be left undigested in the intestines and other parts of the stomach.

This is one myth that has been around for some time and may be part of the argument for some vegetarians and vegans. However, the idea that red meat is just going to sit around undigested in your stomach is silly. Like the other foods that you consume, meat is going to be absorbed in your small intestines before it has time to reach the colon. The idea that meat is able to stay there unabsorbed in the GI tract is just something from the movies.

There are some things in our life that can cause bowel obstruction. But these are going to be things like a physical injury or a disease. Red meat isn't something that is able to block up the GI tract. Because there isn't all that much coming out at the time, those who have smaller bowel movements will assume that all the waste is getting stuck inside of them.

But those smaller movements, including the small movements that happen for those on the carnivore diet, are due to taking in low amounts of fiber. Fiber is going to add in some bulk. When you don't take in the fruits and vegetables, you don't take in the bulk, and this means that your bowel movements are going to be a bit smaller than before.

The good news is that this isn't a bad thing. Your bowel movements will be just fine and you won't notice any constipation or other issues when you go on the carnivore diet. You won't have to get worried about how many bowel movements you are having or whether the red meat is getting stuck inside. Many of those who went on the carnivore diet found that they didn't have any water retention, bloating, or distension when they were on the diet plan. They reported feeling light and like there was more bounce to their step than before starting this diet.

One major concern that can be a problem with the carnivore diet is that it could increase your risk of cancer. There is a lot of evidence out there about how the phytonutrients from plant foods are able to help protect your DNA and keep certain diseases like cancer away. If you are not consuming these plant products, it could affect your long-term health and there are some thoughts that this kind of diet plan could increase your risk of developing cancer.

Bacteria that are in our stomachs, in the GI tract, and in the colon are going to ferment the fiber that we eat into butyrate, a short chain fatty acid. This fatty acid is able to make sure that there is less inflammation in the GI tract, which means that it could be responsible for reducing our risks of colon cancer in the GI tract and more. This is why some experts are against their patients and other individuals going on the carnivore diet.

With that said, there is some research that goes the other way as well. Many people have gone on the ketogenic diet, which is very similar and found that the diet plan was an effective way for them to handle their cancer. Some even found that it could be an effective treatment for chemotherapy and making patients do better during that phase of their treatment. As of right now though, it appears that more evidence is needed to see how things will go with this diet plan over the long term.

It is important to note that while some doctors do believe that going on an all animal diet like this one would increase the risk of colon cancer, it is not because they think animal foods are carcinogenic in any way. The problem is the foods that you take out of the diet, rather than the ones that you put into the diet. You won't be consuming things that can help to inhibit colon cancer. Since you are cutting out these fruits and vegetables so much, it becomes really hard to fight off cancer because the inflammation gets so bad. This doesn't mean that red meat is bad, it just means that you are missing out on some of the things that your body needs in addition to the red meat to stay healthy.

The next concern that some people have with this diet plan is what happens to the gut biome or the balance of bacteria in the stomach that can help you digest food and prevent disease when you go on this kind of diet plan. What was found is that going on an all animal diet had zero effect on the flora, the bad bacteria, when the diet plan was done. And there were usually still higher numbers of the beneficial flora as well.

The reason for this is that the carnivore diet is a good elimination diet. It is going to starve out all of the sugar-hungry bad bacteria until they are all gone because you aren't taking in any carbs or sugars in the process. Yes, this could end up starving out some of the good bacteria as well. But it may be that we don't really need as many of those as we thought. And maybe we only need high levels of those when we are eating a diet that is higher in plant foods. This is something that hasn't been studied in depth yet, but as more people hear about the carnivore diet and how it works, it may be something that more researchers become interested in finding out.

Outside of those who are looking to go on this diet who have some high nutrition needs, or those who need to be careful about how many nutrients they eat because of some medical reasons, the carnivore diet is seen as relatively healthy and it isn't going to lead to many, if any, serious mineral or vitamin deficiencies. As long as the individual follows the diet plan the right way and makes sure that they take in plenty of healthy nutrients, they will find that following this kind of diet plan doesn't have to be as difficult as it may seem.

Just by eating red meat, you are going to take in large amounts of the zinc and iron that the body needs. And the seafood and dairy that you consume are going to have the vitamin D that the body needs, something that usually needs to be added to the plant foods. The one nutrient that can be hard to get ahold of when you aren't eating plants is vitamin C, but there are other ways to get plenty of this nutrient into the body.

When it comes to eating vitamin C though, some supporters of the carnivore diet will talk about how, when you don't take in carbs, you don't actually need as much vitamin C as you do when you consume the produce. This means that even small amounts of vitamin C do well. In fact, there is some speculation that the ketone known as beta-hydroxybutyrate, which your body is going to start producing naturally when you take the carbs out of the diet, can help to replace the need for vitamin C, at least in part.

When you are on a balanced diet, one of the roles of vitamin C is to form collagen, but it is believed that the amino acids that you get from a large meat intake can help you get this job done without needing the produce. And no one who has gone on this diet plan and has come back and reported that they had scurvy, when they went on the carnivore diet, or any of the other similar diet plans that are out there.

The major thing that you need to work on here is to make sure that when you eat the animal foods that are allowed on this diet plan, you make sure that you add in a lot of variety. Don't get stuck on just eating one type of food all of the time. Just like with any diet plan, if you simply eat hamburgers each night and nothing else, you will end up with an issue of not getting enough nutrients into the body. But when you eat enough variety of foods, even with an all-animal-product of the carnivore diet, you will ensure that your body gets the nutrition that it needs to stay healthy.

Missing out on the nutrients

For most people who choose to go on the carnivore diet, you will still be able to get all of the vitamins and nutrients that you need to stay healthy. You will be amazed at how many vitamins and minerals can be found inside of the different sources of meat. While we have been told for years that the only way to get these minerals is through the fruits and vegetables, and sometimes the whole grains that we eat, the truth is that most of these can be found in the protein and animal products that are promoted on this diet plan.

The key here is to eat a lot of variety. If you only eat steak each and every night on this diet plan, it may taste good, but you won't get as much variety in your diet as you should. You need to make sure that you go through all of the different options of animal products to ensure that you are going to get all of the nutrients. Eating a good variety of beef, pork, bacon, turkey, chicken, and fish will ensure that you get all of the nutrients that you could be missing when you cut vegetables and fruits out of your diet.

With that said, there are some people who struggle with getting the nutrients that they need on this diet plan. Often it is because they don't follow it right and get stuck with eating just one type of meat. They don't add variety to their meals and they end up eating the same two or three recipes each day. Without the variety that is needed, it is hard to provide the body with the nutrients that it needs to thrive. When this happens, there could be some complications that arise and this can prove very problematic.

If you are not willing to take the time to find a lot of different recipes that include many different types of animal products, then there could be issues with nutrient deficiency. But this can be true with any diet plan that you choose. The traditional American diet is often going to be full of foods that provide no nutritional value, and even though the participants eat way too many calories, they miss out on the variety and the nutrients that they need and they can deal with a nutrient deficiency as well. Follow the rules of the carnivore diet and make sure that you add as much variety into your animal product choices as possible to keep the body healthy.

Is there anyone who shouldn't go on the carnivore diet?

For the average healthy individual, there is no reason not to go on the carnivore diet. It is completely healthy, as long as you learn how to follow it the proper way and you make sure that you take in the nutrients that are needed. If you can add in lots of variety to keep your nutrient content up, you will be able to lose weight, improve your health, and see some great benefits when you decide to go on the carnivore diet plan.

With that said, there are some people who should not go on the carnivore diet. First, younger children should not go on this kind of diet plan and teenagers should use caution when using it as well. Unless their doctor has prescribed this kind of diet for some reason or another, this diet plan may not be healthy for younger children and teenagers to go on. These age groups need to have a large variety of nutrients, and it is hard for them to get the nutrition that they need from just animal products.

Women who are pregnant or nursing will also need to be careful when it comes to going on the carnivore diet. Just like with the children and teenagers, women who are pregnant or nursing will need more nutrition than they can sometimes get with just animal products, both for themselves and for their babies. If you still feel like the carnivore diet is the right choice for you, make sure to talk this over with your doctor ahead of time so you can see if there are any other health concerns that could occur by following this kind of diet plan.

In addition, if you are dealing with any special health conditions, you may choose to talk to your doctor before you decide to go through with the carnivore diet. There are some health conditions that could be difficult to manage when you do go on this kind of diet plan, and this could make it dangerous for these patients to choose. If you are on any medications for a health condition, always talk with your doctor before you decide to go on this diet plan to ensure that it is safe and healthy for you.

Can athletes go on the carnivore diet?

The ketogenic diet has already taken a lot of heat from critics, and those who believe that if you exercise on a regular basis, you need to have carbs to help your body do well. But over and over again, science has shown that not only is it possible for you to work out even while on a low-carb diet, it is also possible for you to perform at an elite level while on this diet plan.

However, with the carnivore diet, you are taking away all of the plant foods and all of the carbs. The ketogenic diet and other low-carb diets ask you to get rid of most of the carbs, but you are allowed to have some still. With the carnivore diet, your carb intake is going to be almost nothing. This could spell out some differences when it comes to intense workouts and other things that you need to watch out for when you are on this kind of diet plan.

The short answer to this issue is that for right now, we are not certain what the long-term results would be when following the carnivore diet and how it would affect your overall performance, endurance, and muscle mass. With that said, many dieters who are on the carnivore diet will report that even though they were required to reduce their carb intake to almost nothing, they still saw some good gains in muscle mass and endurance overall. In fact, some participants said that they saw much better gains than they had seen in the past on any other diet program.

Now, one thing to remember is that when you switch over from your traditional American diet or another diet plan that requires a lot of carbs to the carnivore diet, you are going to feel worn out and tired in the process. Your body isn't able to get a steady source of carbs and glucose that it is used to, and it can take some time to make adjustments over to relying on fats for fuels. During the first few weeks, you may find that it is beneficial to cut down on the workouts that you do, maybe even stopping them, so that the body has time to rest and adjust, before trying to increase your gains.

In addition, most of the gains were seen with weightlifting and there hasn't been a lot of research into how cardio is going to fair.

Those who do intense cardio may have more trouble with the carnivore diet because fat doesn't convert over to fuel fast enough, in most cases, to deal with cardio and the intense movement that you need to do here. You may need to either cut down on the amount of cardio that you perform or find another way to work out that can help you get stronger, without using the fuel too quickly.

If you are someone who really likes to go hard on your workouts on a frequent basis and if you are an intense athlete, it may be best to make some modifications to the carnivore diet to ensure that you are getting the right kind of nutrition to keep your body moving and to help you see success. But for most people who just exercise on occasion, or who are fine doing some shorter workouts, the traditional carnivore diet is going to help out with this.

How Does Exercise Fit into the Carnivore Diet?

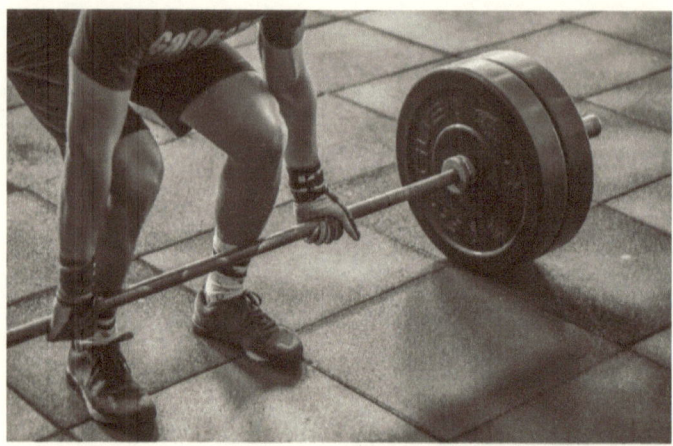

The next thing that we need to take a look at when it comes to the carnivore diet is whether it is acceptable and suitable for those who like to work out. You may wonder whether you need to work out at all when you are on this kind of plan, or if you are going to be able to keep up with your current workout plan when you decide to go on this method. This chapter will take a look at how exercise is going to fit in well with the carnivore diet and explore more about this amazing diet plan as well.

Carnivore Diet and Helping Athletes

One thing that many body lifters have noticed when they go on the ketogenic diet is that their overall performance athletically decreased while they were on this diet plan. Of course, there is the idea that you can work with a targeted ketogenic diet or a cyclical ketogenic diet, but many athletes are choosing to go with the carnivore diet instead to help them reach their overall goals.

There seems to be a rise in athletes who are trying to incorporate a meat only diet into their lives and their workouts, and many of them are seeing some great results. And because of the results that these individuals are seeing, it is likely that as time goes on, this kind of eating could become the standard in the industry.

While the carnivore diet has technically been around for hundreds of years in some form, there still haven't been a lot of studies done to show how this could be the optimal diet when it comes to the performance of athletes. But there is some evidence out there that could point to how successful this kind of diet plan could be for many people.

The idea here is that when you increase the amount of protein that you consume on a daily basis, which is what happens when you go on the carnivore diet, it provides athletes with just enough sugar (which is something that can happen to the protein you eat, thanks to the process of gluconeogenesis) to help increase your performance when you really need to use those smaller amounts of sugars.

This can be great news for a lot of bodybuilders. Often these bodybuilders need a little bit of glucose and maybe some sugars to help them finish out intense workouts and to ensure that they are able to gain more muscle and gain strength. This is why the targeted and cyclical versions of the ketogenic diet were introduced.

But instead of trying to cheat on the carnivore diet and add in those extra sugars and carbs at specific times, you simply just need to make sure that you consume enough protein in your diet and that can then get converted to sugar through the process of gluconeogenesis.

So, instead of hoping to rely on just ketones for energy, like what happens with other low-carb diets, you are able to benefit on the carnivore diet because it will produce small amounts of glucose. This glucose will then be present in your body when you really need it for the anaerobic movements that are so necessary for the weightlifting and bodybuilding field.

Another thing to notice with the carnivore diet is that if you follow the rules of this diet plan strictly, your body is going to have some extra collagen to work with. This collagen can be amazing because it is critical in helping both the joints and the muscles recover after an intense workout. Collagen is going to be the protein source that will bind together everything in your body, from the skin to the joints, and it has to be in abundant supply to make sure that everything inside the body is working in the proper manner.

There are a lot of skeptics out there who believe that the carnivore diet is not healthy or that you should go with one that adds in some carbs, especially fruits and vegetables. We have been told for years that produce, as well as whole grains for that matter, are an important part of our diet. And without them, we are going to feel tired, hungry, and our athletic performance is going to take a hit.

This may be one of the biggest reasons that people won't try out the carnivore diet at all. They worry that they are going to lose out on any of the gains that they have received so far and they don't want that to happen. But the testimonies and the research seem to be against these facts. Instead, when you go on the carnivore diet, it appears that your gains are going to increase. Many people have chosen to go on the carnivore diet and have seen some tremendous results in the process. It is just a matter of getting used to the foods that you need to eat on this diet plan and avoiding issues with cheating along the way.

What about the Cardio

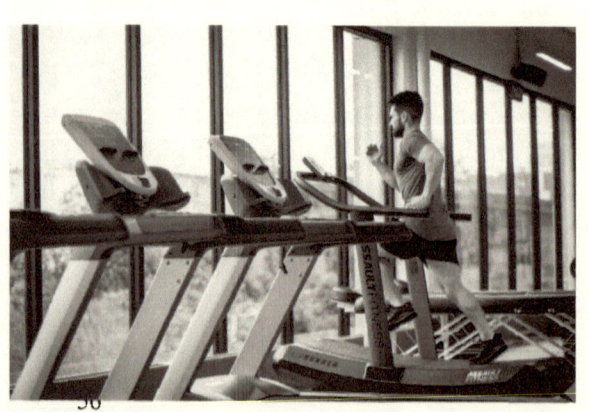

If you are someone who likes to do intense cardio workouts, you may need to cut back on them a little bit. For most people, this is not a problem and you will still be able to add in a bit of cardio to your routine without any issues. But for those who like to do an hour or more of running each day, and who aren't willing to cut it down and take it easy, the carnivore diet may not be the right thing for you to try out.

When you spend a lot of time and energy on cardio each day, you will notice that the body will need an easy source of carbs to help it out. Glucose can be broken down and used quickly, which is what we need to ensure that we can keep going with those longer and harder workouts. While fat can help with the strength training workouts, it can't be converted into energy fast enough to help you get done with the cardio that you need.

If you are someone who likes to do those intense workouts, you may need to take some time to make adjustments to your diet to help you get in some more carbs to your diet right around the workout. Or, you may need to pick out a different type of diet plan to help you with this.

The good news is that most people are not going to need to work out as hard as this in order to get their workout done. This means that they will get the benefit of still being on the carnivore diet and getting to do a bit of cardio. If you keep your cardio levels down and don't go all out all of the time, you will do just fine with this kind of plan.

Another option that you can work on if you would like to do an intense workout while still being on the carnivore diet is to try some HIIT training. HIIT training is known as high-intensity interval training and it allows you to work hard for a minute or so, and then bring the intensity down for five minutes. Doing a few rounds of these can allow you to get a good workout, without overdoing it. Some studies also say that these cycles of up and down are going to be more efficient to help you see results than doing one long and intense workout. Also, it is still going to work great when you are on the carnivore diet.

Can I See Results Without the Workouts?

One thing that is amazing about the carnivore diet is that you will be able to see some results, even if you don't spend a lot of time working out at the gym or even at home. This is vastly different than what you hear about with some of the other diet plans, but the carnivore diet is so efficient that this is true.

The carnivore diet can be incredibly effective all on its own. You are feeding your body a lot of good nutrients that it needs and you are reducing the amount of bad stuff that you eat. When you learn how to reduce the foods you eat to just animal products, you will naturally be able to cut down on the baked goods, the processed foods, and the high sugar foods. Since these are the foods that are the highest in calories, cutting these out means that you will dramatically decrease the number of calories that you take in.

If you learn how to follow this diet plan correctly and only eat when you are hungry, rather than relying on the clock to tell you when it is time to eat, then you will naturally cut down on how much you are eating. Many times, the animal products that you will need to consume on this diet plan are going to be filling, and you may naturally start to take in smaller portions or eat fewer meals overall. This can help you to see some more great results with the state of your overall health.

And finally, the fact that the carnivore diet is putting your body into ketosis is going to help you to lose weight as well. The process of ketosis means that your body has started to rely heavily on the fats that you consume. In fact, this is the only source of energy that your body will receive when it is on this kind of diet plan. The body is very efficient at burning the fat that you consume and the fats that are stored on the body.

As a result, you will be able to lose weight while still maintaining high levels of energy and not feel hungry all the time. Even without a good workout each and every day, you will find that the carnivore diet can help you to lose quite a bit of weight in the process.

Of course, it is better to exercise and get in a good workout a few times a week, no matter how efficient the carnivore diet can be. Your heart and your muscles need to spend some time moving, rather than just sitting on the couch. Also, when you add in a good workout routine with this diet plan, it can do some wonderful things for your health, as well as with the results that you get. Try to spend three to four days doing some kind of workout during the week, whether it is a bit of cardio, a bit of strength training, or some combination. The good news is that with the help of this diet plan, you won't have to spend hours in the gym in order to get those extra results and benefits.

Do I Need To Take It Easy Sometimes?

You may find that you need to take it easy on occasion. Your body may not be ready for the big changes that are going to happen when you go on the carnivore diet, and this can leave you tired and worn out. Instead of pushing yourself and trying to take on too much in the process, it is better to take it easy and allow yourself some time to adjust.

If you are in the first week or two of the carnivore diet, it is best if you can just sit back and relax. This is not the time to really go hard with your workout. Your body has spent so much time adjusting to the diet plan that it was on before, the high levels of glucose that it won't know what to do when you take that glucose away. This can lead to a lot of withdrawal symptoms, moodiness, and you feel really tired.

In addition, if you were someone who suffered from sugar addiction before you started on this kind of diet plan, you really need to give yourself a break. Not only are you going to be dealing with the withdrawal issues of glucose and all of the lack of energy and other issues that come from the body not having an easy and steady source of energy, but you will also have to deal with sugar withdrawals.

This is why you should consider taking it easy during the first few weeks that you are on this kind of diet plan. You can try to take a week or so off from work or at least schedule it during a time when you shouldn't be as busy. Take a break from doing your workout routine and just allow yourself to relax, go to bed early, and even nap if you need.

After those first few weeks are done, you will find that your levels of energy start to come back. You will get the benefit of relying on healthy fats to keep you going, which will provide you with a ton more energy than you could have gotten on your traditional eating plan. It just takes some time for the body to switch over and start using the fat source as fuel, so give yourself some time.

Tips to Make the Carnivore Diet More Successful

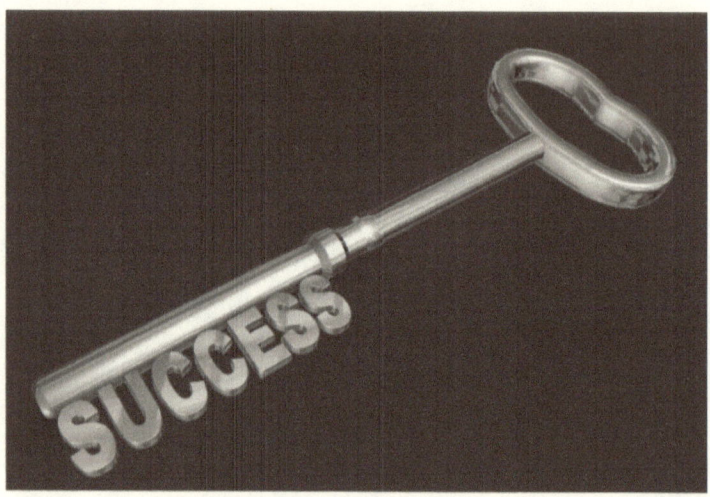

There is so much out there that you can love when it comes to the carnivore diet. It is simple to follow because you only have to remember a few types of foods and not even a lot of food groups in order to know what you are allowed to eat and what you should avoid. It is efficient because if you add in a lot of variety, you will still be able to get all of the vitamins and minerals that the body needs to stay healthy, without all of the bad stuff that you need to avoid for your health. Also, it is going to taste good. If you are already a meat lover, then this is definitely the diet plan for you to choose.

With that said, going on the carnivore diet is going to be a bit different than what you are used to in the past. Whether you have gone on a diet plan in the past or not, the carnivore diet is seen as a more restrictive kind of diet plan compared to some of the others. The good news is there are a lot of tips and tricks that you can follow in order to get the best results with this plan and they include:

Go on the diet plan with a friend

Going on any kind of diet plan can be a challenge. But when it comes to the carnivore diet, you are asked to reduce your eating to just a few types of foods. You are allowed to eat all of the meats that you want, especially fatty meats, eggs, and some dairy products, such as cream, butter, and cheese. But outside of this, you will need to eliminate all of the other food groups. For those who have been on bad eating habits in the past, especially those who have a love for bread and pasta, this can be hard.

Finding a friend to go on this kind of diet plan with you can really make a difference. Both of you will go through the same things while on this diet plan, which means you can be there for each other. You can motivate each other to keep working towards the goal, call each other for support when necessary, share recipes, and so much more.

Don't try to go on the carnivore diet all on your own. Consider finding a friend or even a support group online who can be there to help you get this diet plan done the right way.

Slowly start to eliminate the foods

For some people, the carnivore diet is going to work best if they just go cold turkey. They choose a day that they want to get started with this diet plan and then they go all out with it. On that chosen day, they eliminate most of the dairy, all of the grains, and all of the produce. And of course, they eliminate the amount of processed and baked goods that they are allowed to enjoy as well.

These people find that if they cheat even a little or if they go slowly into the diet plan, they are going to run into trouble. They may have a hard time controlling themselves and won't be able to stop once they have started. For these individuals, it is often best to just jump right in and not look back, otherwise, they will end up failing.

For others, jumping all the way end right from the beginning can be too hard. Maybe they are worried about how their health is going to do if they try to eliminate all of those food groups all at once. Or maybe they want to just ease into it so they don't provide such a shock on their bodies in the process. No matter the reason, it is fine to start eliminating foods slowly.

If you are worried about jumping right in and giving up all of your favorite foods all at once, a better option could be to slowly eliminate the foods. You can start out by just eliminating one food group at a time each week until you are down to the carnivore diet. Others have found that starting out with the ketogenic diet and then slowly moving over when they are ready can help as well.

Relax during the adjustment time

During the first week or two that you are on the carnivore diet, you need to take a break and just relax. Even if you are really excited to lose weight and see results, you still need to take it easy. You will find that starting on the carnivore diet is hard, and sometimes you are going to feel tired and worn out. Going all out with the diet plan and jumping into it too quickly can make you more tired and can make it harder to stick with the diet plan.

The best thing that you can do when you first go on this kind of diet plan is to take it easy. It is never a good idea to jump on this kind of diet plan when you have a busy week, or there are a lot of stressful things that are going on in your life. You want to make sure that you can take it easy when you are on this diet plan, especially in the beginning, and that you don't have a really big project or a lot of work going on at the same time.

If you are able to take an off for a week or so, this could be best. This will allow you to rest, take naps, and not overdo it or feel too stressful when it comes to the work and activities that you need to get done during that time. If you aren't able to do so, see if you are able to limit the amount of work you have to handle during that time. If you can, wait until after a big project is done, or see if you can work from home.

The truth is, while there are a ton of benefits to this diet plan and it is going to help you feel amazing, the first week is going to be tough. Your body is adjusting to a new source of fuel. You have to cut out a lot of your favorite foods, even ones that you had seen as healthy before. Also, you are going to go through a lot of cravings and missing those carbs and sugars. This is all going to come together to make you grumpy, moody, and really tired.

With all of these changes in your emotions and how you feel, it is probably best to not add in too much work or too much stress to make it work. You can see why it may be better to finish up that big project at work first or wait until things slow down, or take time off and work from home, so that you can recover and get adjusted to the new diet plan in a way that keeps you away from others and gives you plenty of rest.

Stay hydrated

Another thing that you may want to consider watching out for when you go on this kind of diet plan is to drink plenty of water. Many times when people go on a low-carb diet, but especially when they go on the carnivore diet, there is an issue with not drinking enough. You may find that you aren't as hungry and then you forget to drink enough water along the way as well.

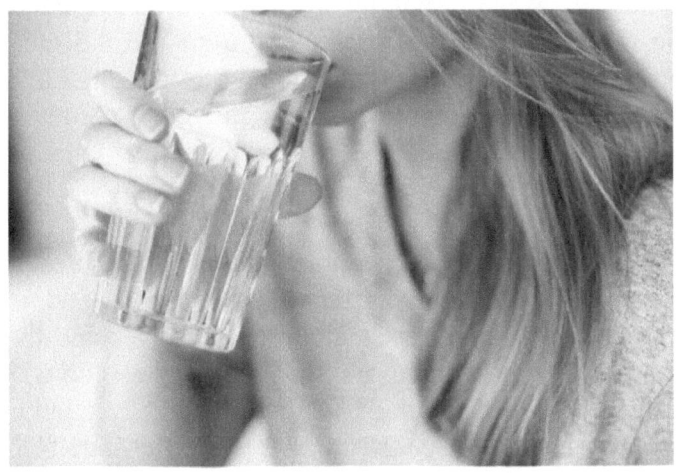 Dehydration is going to make the first few weeks worse and can make the moodiness, cravings, and more a lot harder to deal with. But any time on this diet plan when you aren't taking in enough hydration, you will start to feel miserable. Your body needs this hydration to feel good, to keep in good working shape, and to make sure that you are able to function like normal.

If you find that it is hard to keep hydrated enough on this diet plan, there are options to take. Get a special water bottle that is just for yourself and keep it right next to you during the day. Or each hour, set an alarm that will remind you to take another drink of water, maybe eight ounces each hour or more if you find that you need it. You will be amazed at how much of a difference just drinking a cup or so of water can do for how good you feel while on this diet plan.

Realize that this is going to take some time

Getting used to the carnivore diet can take some time. You may be ready and motivated right off the bat and excited to see the results. But the truth is, the carnivore diet can be a bit difficult to get on. Many people, when they first get started at least, are going to focus on all of the foods that they aren't allowed to have. This can bring them down and make them feel bad. When they look back on all of the foods that they aren't allowed to consume, it can seem a bit overwhelming.

Adjusting to this new way of thinking and getting used to the idea of not being able to consume all the produce, the grains, and other products that you were used to in your traditional diet can be tough. While there are a ton of healthy and tasty foods and animal products that you can eat on the carnivore diet, it does take some time to adjust to this new way of eating.

Being easy on yourself and understanding that this is a process and a lifetime change can make it easier. Sometimes we end up placing too many restrictions and expectations on ourselves and this can be our downfall. We think that we should be able to keep up with the changes right from the start. We think that we should never fall or fail. But we are all human, and the carnivore diet is a big change from what we are used to eating.

When we take it easy on ourselves and we realize that there may be times when we fall off the diet plan, it is going to be much easier to see the results that we want. And if you do end up falling off the wagon and cheating on the diet, don't beat yourself up about it. Just realize that you made a mistake, try to figure out what caused you to make that cheat so you can avoid it next time, and then move on with more determination and a better understanding the next time that you try the diet plan.

Don't exercise in the beginning

During the first few weeks of being on the carnivore diet, you are going to feel really worn down. Your body is not used to not having the carbs and sugars to convert for glucose and help you gain the energy that you need. While the body is going to be just fine switching over to fats as a fuel source, it is going to take some time before this happens.

With that said, you will find that it takes a bit of time before the body is able to switch. During that time, which can vary between one to two weeks depending on that person, you are going to feel worn out and tired. Your body basically feels like it isn't getting the fuel that it needs, even though you are providing it with plenty. You may find that just getting through the regular things that you need to get done during the day can be a difficult task to work on.

During this time, it may not be the best idea to add exercise into the routine. You are going to be worn out enough for a bit. Adding in some workouts can make it even more difficult during this time. If you feel up to it, doing some light weights or going on a walk around the block can help you to keep moving and keeps the blood flowing. But it is much better if you can wait a few weeks before you decide to get on an intense workout program.

Don't worry though. Your body will adjust to using the fats for a fuel source. Once you do, your energy levels are going to go through the roof. You will be impressed by the muscle gains that you can make with weight training and the energy that you have to work with some of the other types of workouts. But before you can get to that point, you need to take it slow and get the body adjusted to these changes.

Find ways to mix up your exercises

When you are on the carnivore diet, you will need to spend some time getting in a few good workouts. You may not want to go as hard during the first few weeks as you did during some of the workouts that you did in the past, but it is certainly fine for you to spend some time working out to look and feel better. The carnivore diet is going to be so much more effective when you take the time to work out.

Many people find that they get in a rut with working out though because they only do one kind all of the time. They like to spend their time weight lifting, or doing cardio, or doing some stretches like Yoga, and they never mix it up and try new things.

If you would really like to improve your strength and endurance, and you want to make sure that you really see some great results, you need to make sure that you are mixing up the types of workouts that you are going to do. Doing a bit of strength training, a bit of cardio, and a bit of stretching can do some wonders when you want to lose weight and help you to feel better.

Let's start with eight training. You will want to spend a few days a week on this, even if you don't want to really see some gains in muscle tone. Those who aren't body lifters are able to make sure that they get lean and lose more weight if they add on a bit of weight to the workout, and concentrate on some of the different muscle groups to see results.

Next is the cardio. You don't want to go too crazy with the cardio that you are doing on the carnivore diet. Since you aren't using carbs with your diet on this plan, you may find that you aren't able to convert the fat over to a usable fuel source quick enough. But doing some light cardio two to three days a week will make a big difference, and is perfectly doable when you are on this kind of diet plan.

You can also spend some time working on your stretching. This will ensure that you are able to relax the muscles and can prevent injuries. You can just do some basic stretches, or you can choose to do something like Yoga to help you get the same results.

Find ways to distract yourself when the cravings occur

There are going to be times when those cravings start to get to you. This is especially true if you are dealing with the first few weeks of being on this kind of diet plan. You will find that your body craves the sugars and the carbs, and the fact that you kicked them out of your diet in a short amount of time can make it even harder to make the adjustments that you would like.

If you are just sitting around the house and not doing anything, you will keep thinking about the cravings and avoiding the cravings is going to seem almost impossible. The longer that you keep yourself at home and not doing anything, the harder it is going to be to avoid the cravings. And if you continue to sit around the house, it is likely that you are going to give in to the cravings and lose some of the results that you are getting with this plan.

The best thing that you can do when it is time to avoid the cravings that you are going to deal with is to find ways to distract yourself. There are a lot of things that you can do to make sure that you are easily distracted and won't give in to some of those cravings. You can choose to go on a walk around the block, do a good workout, clean the house, read a book, go out with some friends, and more. The important thing here is to do something that gets your mind off the foods and the cravings that you have, and avoid giving in and losing the results that you want to get with this diet plan.

Remember what your motivation is

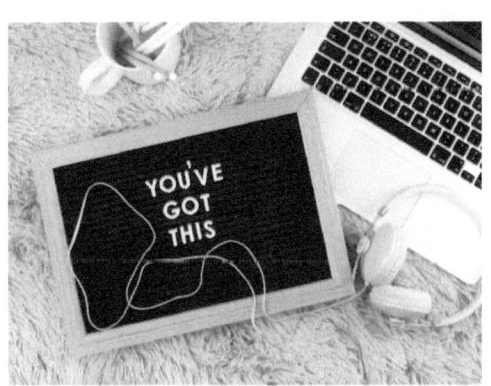

The carnivore diet is going to be hard sometimes. While it would be nice to find out that you could eat whatever you want and lose weight or to find a diet plan that wouldn't cause you any troubles or roadblocks, this is just not reality. And in truth, the carnivore diet does ask you to give up a lot of the foods that you know and love.

The cravings are going to be hard, the low energy in the beginning is going to be hard, and when you see others around you enjoying pasta and other foods that you love, it is sometimes going to be hard to stick with your goals. But the best way for you to deal with this new diet plan is to find the right motivation to keep you going.

Before you even get started on this diet plan, you should take some time to figure out what your motivation is all about. This is going to be the thing that will keep you going, even when things get tough. Maybe you are looking to lose weight and fit back into some of your clothes after having a baby or just letting yourself go a bit. Maybe you want to get the endurance to run a marathon, or you want to be able to have better health and get off some of your medications.

No matter what your own personal motivation is to start with, you need to set this up ahead of time and make sure that you stick with it for the long-term. This is something that you can take a look back at later on, to ensure that you will stick with the diet, no matter how tough it gets. And there are going to be some times when things do get tough and you will need a pick-up. With the right motivation, you will get that pick-up and get back on track in no time.

Find some good recipes to make this plan easier

One of the hardest things that you will run into when you get started on the carnivore diet is that you aren't sure what kinds of foods you are allowed to consume. There are a lot of restrictions when

70

it comes to this particular diet plan. You may have looked through some of the foods that are allowed (and the long list of foods that are not allowed) for this diet plan and then wondered how you were going to find the right recipes to make this happen.

Once you stop concentrating on all of the foods that you are not allowed to have, and instead find ways to concentrate on all of the good foods you are allowed to have, this diet plan is going to seem so much easier. Think of it this way, you get to enjoy all of the hamburgers, steaks, ribs, and other great meat sources that you want when you are on this diet plan. What could be better than that!

Sometimes it is hard to get started on this diet plan because of the recipes. This guidebook is going to provide you with a lot of tasty recipes that you are sure to enjoy without feeling deprived. We will have recipes that work for breakfast, lunch, dinner, and sides and appetizers, and they include all of the tasty meat and eggs that you could ever dream about. After you are on this diet plan for a short amount of time, you will find that it is easier than ever to find some of your new favorite recipes to help you lose weight and get in the best health possible.

The carnivore diet is a great choice to go on. It can help you to lose weight and get in the best health of your life. But sometimes, it is going to be a challenge to get on this diet plan and stick with it. Compared to most of the other diet plans out there, it is going to be a lot harder. It has simple ideas and you only have to remember a few things to be successful in it. But since you are giving up some of your favorite foods in the process, you may worry about whether you can make it through.

If you are able to follow some of the tips and suggestions that are in this chapter, then you will find that the carnivore diet doesn't have to be as hard as it may seem. With some patience and some time, you will find that you are going to see a lot of results when you go on this kind of diet plan.

21-Day Meal Plan for the Carnivore Diet

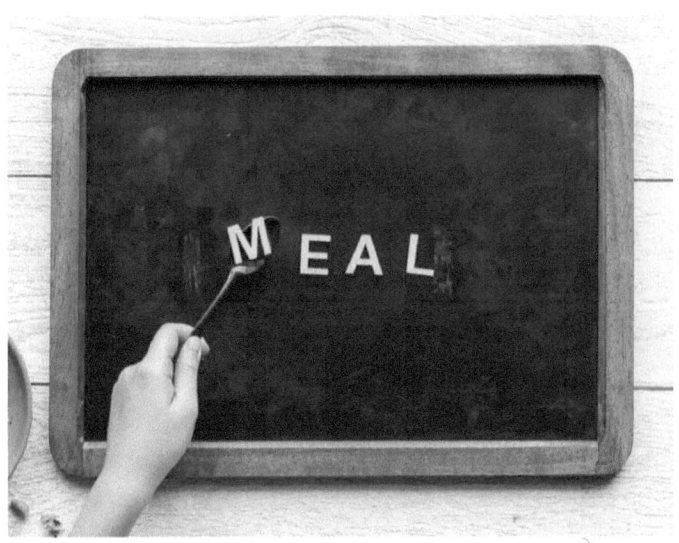

Sometimes the hardest thing to deal with when you get started on a new diet plan is figuring out which meals you should make. The carnivore diet can take some extra planning to accomplish because it does limit the foods that you get to eat. And while it may seem pretty simple to figure out, when you come home at the end of the day, you may be worried about what you should cook for dinner that day, or what you should deal with when it comes to lunchtime.

Figuring out the meals that you are going to eat during the first few weeks on this diet plan can be sometimes difficult. The rest of this guidebook is going to take some time to provide you with a 21-day meal plan for the carnivore diet plan, as well as information on the recipes and how to make each one. As you can see, there are a lot of great meals that you can enjoy while on this diet plan and still get all the nutrition and variety that you are looking for while following this kind of plan.

Day 1:	Day 2:	Day 3:
Breakfast: *Poached Eggs* **Lunch:** *Fried Chicken Hearts* **Dinner:** *Slow Cooker Pulled Pork*	**Breakfast:** *Grilled Beef Patties* **Lunch:** *Baked Chicken Thighs* **Dinner:** *Chicken and Pork Rind*	**Breakfast:** *Sliced Cold Beef* **Lunch:** *BBQ Trout* **Dinner:** *Bacon and Shredded Chicken*
Day 4:	Day 5:	Day 6:
Breakfast: *Sous Vide Recipe* **Lunch:** *Smoked Lamb Ribs* **Dinner:** *Southern Steak*	**Breakfast:** *Baked Eggs with Cream* **Lunch:** *Skinny Steaks* **Dinner:** *Roasted Cream Chicken and Bone Broth*	**Breakfast:** *Bacon and Chorizo Sausage Bake* **Lunch:** *Salami Crisps* **Dinner:** *Pan Roasted Duck Breasts*
Day 7:	Day 8:	Day 9:
Breakfast: *Breakfast Meatloaf* **Lunch:** *Slow-Baked Salmon* **Dinner:** *Pork tenderloin on the Stove*	**Breakfast:** *Chicken Liver Pate* **Lunch:** *Broiled Flank Steak* **Dinner:** *Roasted Turkey*	**Breakfast:** *Poached Eggs* **Lunch**: *Beef Chuck Roast* **Dinner:** *Slow Cooker Beef Tongue*

Day 10:	Day 11:	Day 12:
Breakfast: *Breakfast Meatloaf* **Lunch:** *Beef Roast with Bone Broth* **Dinner:** *Oyster Cream Panfry*	**Breakfast:** *Grilled Beef Patties* **Lunch:** *Reverse Sear Steak* **Dinner:** *Steamed Clams or Mussels*	**Breakfast:** *Sous Vide Recipe* **Lunch:** *T-bone Grilled Steak* **Dinner:** *Chicken Livers Wrapped in Bacon*
Day 13:	Day 14:	Day 15:
Breakfast: *Sliced Cold Beef* **Lunch:** *Fried Chicken Hearts* **Dinner:** *Slow Cooker Chicken Gizzards*	**Breakfast:** *Baked Eggs with Cream* **Lunch:** *Baked Chicken Thighs* **Dinner:** *Slow Cooker Pulled Pork*	**Breakfast:** *Poached Egg* **Lunch:** *BBQ Trout* **Dinner:** *Chicken and Pork Rind*
Day 16:	Day 17:	Day 18:
Breakfast: *Bacon and Chorizo Sausage Bake* **Lunch:** *Smoked Lamb Ribs* **Dinner:** *Southern Steak*	**Breakfast:** *Chicken Liver Pate* **Lunch:** *Salami Crisps* **Dinner:** *Pan Roasted Duck Breasts*	**Breakfast:** *Breakfast Meatloaf* **Lunch:** *Skinny Steaks* **Dinner:** *Roasted Cream Chicken and Bone Broth*

Day 19:	Day 20:	Day 21:
Breakfast:	**Breakfast:**	**Breakfast:**
Baked Eggs with Cream	*Grilled Beef Patties*	*Bacon and Chorizo Sausage Bake*
Lunch:	**Lunch:**	**Lunch:**
Slow-Baked Salmon	*Broiled Flank Steak*	*Beef Chuck Roast*
Dinner:	**Dinner:**	**Dinner:**
Roasted Turkey	*Oyster Cream Panfry*	*Steamed Clams or Mussels*

Easy Breakfasts on the Carnivore Diet

The first meal of the day can often be the most important. When it is time to sit down and enjoy a nice breakfast, you will find that there are still lots of options. This is a great time to enjoy some of the leftovers that you may have from the night before or make a new creation. Eggs are the perfect thing to enjoy if you want something simple and quick to start out your morning, but some of these great options can work as well!

Poached Eggs

What's inside:

Eggs (2)
Salt (.5 tsp.)
Butter (3 tbsp.)

How to make:

1. To start this recipe, bring out a skillet and heat it up a bit. Add in the butter and let it heat up for the next minute until soft.
2. At this time, gently crack the eggs, making sure that the yolks stay intact when you place them in the pan.
3. Sprinkle some salt over the eggs and then cook the eggs until they are all done to your liking.
4. Take the skillet off the heat, place the eggs on a plate, and enjoy.

Grilled Beef Patties

What's inside:

Aged Swiss cheese (8 slices)
Salt (.5 tsp.)
Melted lard (1 tbsp.)
Ground beef (2 lbs.)

For the fried eggs
Free range eggs (8)
Butter (2 Tbsp.)

How to make:

1. To start this recipe, combine together the salt, melted lard, and ground beef, mixing together lightly.
2. Once those are done, you can take the meat and shape it into eight patties that are pretty even.
3. Turn on the grill and get it hot. Once it is warmed up, add the eight patties to the grill and let them cook.
4. You will want the internal temperature of the meat to be around 160 degrees. This can take grilling about seven minutes on each side.
5. Now you can work on the eggs. You can bring out two large skillets. Take a tablespoon of the butter and melt it on each one while heating them on the grill.
6. Break four eggs into a saucer and then gently slide them into your pans. Reduce the heat to low. Try to place the eggs with the sunny side up and then cover the pan.
7. These need to cook for four minutes so that the yolks start to thicken, but they don't get hard. If you would like to work with basted eggs, smear a bit of extra butter over them as you continue to cook.
8. Flip the eggs around until all of the sides are cooked properly. Place the Swiss cheese on top of each egg until they start to melt. Serve the eggs on top of the burger patties and enjoy.

Sliced Cold Beef

What's inside:

Melted butter or ghee (1 tbsp.)
Salt
Cross rib roast (2 lb.)

How to make:

1. Take the roast out of the fridge and let it sit for half an hour to an hour to warm up a bit and to ensure nice and even cooking.
2. After this time has passed, you can turn on the oven and let it heat up to 250 degrees.
3. While the oven is heating up, you can take the beef and season it with some salt all over. Then pour the melted ghee or butter on top to coat the beef lightly.
4. Put the beef into a baking dish or a roasting pan. Place the pan into the oven and give it time to heat up.
5. After 2 hours, take the meat out of the oven and check the temperature. Once it reaches 130 degrees, the meat will be medium rare. Cook for a bit longer if you want a different level of doneness.
6. Allow the beef to cool down on the counter for half an hour. Add to the fridge to cool down completely before slicing and serving.

Sous Vide Recipe

What's inside:

Ghee (1.5 tbsp.)
Salt
Eye of the round roast (3 lbs.)

How to make:

1. Take out a sous vide and fill it with some water. Set it to reach 140 degrees.
2. Bring out a FoodSaver bag and place the roast inside along with a tablespoon of ghee. Vacuum seal the bag and place it in the fridge until the sous vide is warmed up
3. Once your sous vide reaches the right temperature, you can place the vacuum-sealed beef inside and let it cook for some time.
4. After 24 hours, take the meat out of the bag and pat it dry using some paper towels.
5. Take the rest of the ghee and heat it on a skillet. Season the eye of the round with some salt and place it into the warmed up skillet.
6. Sear the meat on all sides for about 60 seconds each side. Take the meat out of the skillet and let it rest before slicing up and serving.

Baked Eggs with Cream

What's inside:

Salt
Eggs (2)
Heavy whipping cream (2 tbsp.)
Softened butter (.5 tbsp.)

How to make:

1. Heat up the oven and give it some time to reach 425 degrees. While the oven is heating up, take out a four-ounce ramekin and coat it all over with some butter.
2. Add the cream into the ramekin and then crack the eggs into it as well. Add this to the oven to bake.
3. After about 10 minutes, the whites of the eggs should be done. Take the eggs out and then serve warm.

Bacon and Chorizo Sausage Bake

What's inside:

Bacon, cooked (3 slices)
Salt
Eggs (2)
Chorizo sausage (4 oz.)
Butter (1 tsp.)
Lard or tallow (2 tbsp.)

How to make:

1. Turn on the oven and give it some time to heat up to 350 degrees. While the oven is heating up, use the butter to prepare two ramekins for this recipe.
2. Take out a skillet and heat up your lard or your tallow inside. This needs to heat up for three minutes to make soft.
3. Chop up the chorizo sausage in the pan until it is done. When the sausage is done, divide it into equal amounts in each of the ramekins.
4. Slowly crack your egg into each ramekin and then season with some salt. Place into the oven to bake.
5. After 13 minutes, the dish should be done. Take it out of the oven before topping with the bacon and serving.

Breakfast Meatloaf

What's inside:

Beef, ground (.5 lb.)
Salt
Lard
Bacon strips (4)
Parmesan cheese (1 c.)
Egg (1)
Butter (3 tbsp.)
Ground pork (.5 lb.)

How to make:

1. To start this recipe, turn on the oven and let it heat up to 350 degrees.
2. While the oven is warming up, take out a bowl and mix together salt, parmesan cheese, egg, beef, and ground pork. Make sure that the mixture sticks together.
3. Use this mixture to form two small logs and then individually tie them up with bacon strips starting from the top. Use as many bacon strips as you need for this.
4. Add the butter to a pan and then turn the heat on a high setting. When the butter is melted, you can place the meatloaf in, allowing the bacon seam to face down to avoid spillage.
5. Flip and cook the meat on both sides to make it browned. After the meat is browned, add the meat to a pan and place into the oven.
6. After 15 minutes of cooking, take the meatloaf out and allow it to rest a bit. Slice this up and serve warm.

Chicken Liver Pate

What's inside:

Butter (.5 c.)
Chicken liver (.5 lb.)
Rosemary sprig
Pepper
Salt
Double cream (2 tbsp.)

How to make:

1. Bring out a frying pan and melt a tablespoon of butter inside. When the butter is nice and melted, you can add in the chopped liver and let it cook for eight minutes.
2. After this time, you can add the liver into the food processor. Add the leftover butter from the pan and some cheese as well.
3. Melt the rosemary, salt, pepper, thyme, and two more tablespoons of the butter together. When those are smooth, add them into the food processor with the liver.
4. Blend the liver in the food processor at this time until it is smooth. Pour the mixture into some ramekins.
5. Melt the rest of the butter that you have on the stove. Then cover the pate with it and add some rosemary leaves on top.
6. Make sure to add this to the fridge to chill a bit before serving.

Lunches to Keep the Hunger Away

The next thing that we need to take a look at is the tasty lunches that can make or break your day. In the middle of the day, after working or playing hard so far today, you will want to make sure that you can have something that is tasty and easy to make. No one has the time to work on a meal that will take over an hour or more to make, but you want to make sure that you get to enjoy something that is tasty and healthy for you. Some of the tasty meals that you can enjoy on your lunch break, even on a leisurely weekend and are carnivore-friendly include:

Fried Chicken Hearts

What's inside:

Chicken hearts, quartered (500 g.)
Butter (2 tbsp.)
Fish sauce or salt to taste

How to make:

1. Take out a frying pan and heat up some of the butter inside until it has time to melt.
2. Once the butter melts, you can add in the chicken hearts. Stirring them around the whole time, cook these until they brown. Then cover the frying pan.
3. Reduce the heat to a low setting now and let the chicken hearts cook until the pink center is gone. This can take around 15 minutes to be done.
4. Add in some of the fish sauce or some salt and then cover the pan again. Cook for an additional five minutes before serving hot.

Baked Chicken Thighs

What's inside:

Salt
Chicken thighs (4)

How to make:

1. To start this recipe, turn on the oven and give it time to heat up to 400 degrees.
2. Bring out a baking dish or a baking pan and add the chicken thighs to it. Season these chicken thighs with some salt before placing into the preheated oven.
3. Allow these to bake for a bit. This is going to take about 30 minutes to bake or go until the pink coloration that is in the bones starts to run clear.
4. After this time, take the pan out of the oven and serve hot.

BBQ Trout

What's inside:

Salt
Wild sea trout (6 lbs.)

How to make:

1. To start this recipe, scale the wild trout, take the gills, eyes, and guts out and then wash it off. Pat dry with a kitchen towel all over to make sure that there are no running drips.
2. Take the fish and make some diagonal cuts on the sides. Sprinkle a bit of salt into these cuts.
3. Bring out some newspapers and wrap the trout up in multiple layers to ensure that it is sealed right. Use butchers string to help secure the newspapers.
4. Submerge the trout in the papers in cold water. This is meant to help get the newspaper wet a little bit.
5. Turn on the grill and let it heat up. Add the fish into it and cook for about forty minutes. You can occasionally flip this around until it is ready.
6. After this time, you can take the fish off the grill and allow it time to cool down for a few minutes.
7. Cut off the string and remove the newspaper that was around the fish. Place the fish on a tray and flake off the fish with a fork. Enjoy the fish right away.

Smoked Lamb Ribs

What's inside:

Butter (1 tbsp.)
Lamb rib chops (8)
Pepper
Salt (1 Tbsp.)

How to make:

1. Take out the lamb chops and rub pepper and salt all over it to start this recipe.
2. Turn on the smoker and get it set up for indirect heating. When you are ready, you can add the ribs onto the cooler part of the smoker so that they don't come in direct contact with the fire.
3. Cover the smoker and let these go for a bit. After an hour, take the ribs out and wrap them up with some foil.
4. Place them back into the smoker, letting the meat side be down, and continue to cook for another bit.
5. After another 35 minutes, you can flip these around and cook for another half an hour to finish.
6. Once this time is up, take the ribs from the smoker and give them half an hour to cool down.
7. Unwrap the ribs at this point and then serve.

Skinny Steaks

What's inside:

Sliced beef sirloin (2 lbs.)
Pepper
Salt

How to make:

1. Take your fatty beef strip and season it with the pepper and salt. Then place it in the fridge to set with the seasonings for the next two hours or so.
2. After this time is up, take the steak out of the fridge and pat it dry with the help of some paper towels.
3. Turn on the grill as high as you can get it, but leave the lid open. If you are using a charcoal grill, make sure that the coals are high enough to do this. If you are using a gas grill, lower the grate so that it is closer to your burner for this meal.
4. Add the meat to the hottest part of the grill. Flip it around to cool the hot surfaces, reduce the heat build-up, and to prevent the inside of the meat from overcooking.
5. You want to get the inside of the meat to 130 degrees, with a middle uniform and dark exterior with no grill marks.
6. Once it reaches the right internal temperature, you can take the steak off the grill and enjoy.

Salami Crisps

What's inside:

Salami slices (12)

How to make:

1. Turn on the oven and let it have time to heat up to 325 degrees.
2. While the oven is warming up, take out a baking sheet and place a piece of parchment paper on the sheet.
3. Arrange the slices of salami out on the baking sheet, making sure that they are in one single layer. Add this to the oven and let it bake.
4. After about ten minutes, the edges of the salami should start to curl up a bit. You can take them out of the oven and allow them some time to cool down before serving.

Slow Baked Salmon

What's inside:

Whole salmon fillet (3 lbs.)
Salt
Melted   butter   or   ghee   (3   Tbsp.)

How to make:

1. Take the salmon out of the fridge and leave it on the counter a bit. We want to let it get a bit closer to room temperature here, so leave it out for half an hour or so.
2. After this half an hour has passed, turn on the oven and give it time to heat up to 275 degrees.
3. Next, take out the salmon and season it with some salt. Spread the butter or the ghee over the salmon as well, and then place it on a baking sheet.
4. Place the salmon into the preheated oven to heat up for a bit. After 30 minutes, check to see how warm the salmon is.
5. If the salmon reaches 120 degrees, you can take it out of the oven, and serve warm.

Broiled Flank Steak

What's inside:

Melted ghee (1 tbsp.)
Salt (.5 tsp.)
Flank steak (1.5 lbs.)

How to make:

1. Take the steak out and let it set on the counter for a bit. After 45 minutes, some of the chill from the fridge should be gone and you can start the recipe. This time is important because it ensures the cooking is even.
2. Add the rack to the top of your oven so that when you add the steak in, it will only be a few inches or less from the broiler.
3. Turn the oven on to broil and let it have some time to heat up.
4. While the oven is warming up, get a baking tray and nestle a wire cooling rack on top of it. Season the steak with some salt and then pour the ghee on top, making sure to spread it all over the top.
5. Place this prepared steak on your cooling rack that is on the baking tray and add it to the oven to bake.
6. Broil the steak for a bit. After four minutes, you can flip the steak around and let it broil a bit longer.
7. After another 6 minutes, check to make sure that the internal temperature of the steak is at least 125 degrees.
8. After the steak has reached the right internal temperature, you can take it out of the oven and give it about five minutes to cool down. Slice the steak into strips and then serve.

Beef Chuck Roast

What's inside:

Shredded parmesan cheese
Bone broth or water (4 c.)
Salt
Chuck roast, bone-in (4 lbs. or more)

How to make:

1. Take the roast out and let it set on the counter for 60 minutes or so to help remove the chill that it gets from being in the fridge and to help you get a more even cooking.
2. When that time is done, turn on the oven and let it heat up to 200 degrees. Slice up the roast into quarters and then season it well with salt. Put the broth and the seasoned beef.
3. Do not put the lid on top of the Dutch oven as you place it into the oven. Cook for a while so the broth and the meat reach 120 degrees.
4. After two hours, you can cover the pot and increase the temperature of the oven up to 250 degrees.
5. Cook this dish for another three to four hours. After that time is done, you can test the meat for tenderness. If it needs a bit longer, go at twenty to thirty-minute intervals here
6. Once the meat is all done, you can take it out of the oven and give it some time to cool down first.
7. Top the individual servings with some of the Parmesan if you would like and serve.

Beef Roast with Bone Broth

What's inside:

Water or bone broth (2 c.)
Salt
Chuck roast (4 lbs.)

How to make:

1. Take the roast out of the fridge and give it 60 minutes or so to warm up a little bit. This helps to get the chill out of the meat and can ensure even cooking.
2. When this time is up, you can quarter up the chuck roast and take the time to generously season it with salt.
3. Take out your Instant Pot and pour the bone broth into the bottom. Add the beef and then secure the lid on tight.
4. Cook the beef on high pressure for about 55 minutes. After that time, you can use the natural release method to let the pressure out.
5. Once all of the pressure is out of the pot, you can take the beef out of the pot and shred it up before serving.

Reverse Sear Steak

What's inside:

Animal fat to help with searing
Sea salt
Steak

How to make:

1. Take out the steak and let it set on the counter for about 45 minutes so that it has time to reach room temperature.
2. Season the steak with some salt. Bring out your baking pan and add a wire cooling rack inside of it. When this is organized, you can place the steak on top.
3. Turn on the oven and give it time to heat up to 275 degrees. When the oven is warm enough, you can add the steak inside to bake.
4. After 40 minutes have passed, you can take the steak out of the oven. Heat up the skillet to high heat and add a bit of the animal fat, such as bacon fat or ghee.
5. When those are warm, you can add in the steak and let it sear on each side for a minute, or until the desired temperature is reached.

T-bone grilled steak

What's inside:

Salt (2 tbsp.)
T-bone steaks (5)

For the rub
Coriander seeds (2 tbsp.)
Cayenne pepper (1 tsp.)
Garlic powder (1 tsp.)
Onion powder (1 tbsp.)

How to make:

1. Take out a small bowl and mix together all of the dry spices, grinding them together if needed.
2. Take out the steaks and rub it all over with salt, getting enough on for your taste.
3. Place the prepared steaks into the fridge and let them marinate and chill there for one to four hours.
4. After this time, heat up the grill and then, once it is hot, place the steaks on and cook them. You can flip the steaks over every two minutes to make sure that both sides get done.
5. After you flip the meat a few times, check the meat temperature. If you want it medium rare, the internal temperature should be about 125 degrees. Cook until it reaches your desired doneness.

Dinners for the Caveman in the Family

And now it is time for the main event! Supper can be an important part of your family getting together and getting to spend time together. After a long day at work and school and all of the other activities that we need to get done during the day, it is nice to come home to a great meal that tastes good and is good and healthy for us. The recipes below will help you to get your meal on the table in no time and still allows you to lose weight and improve your health, thanks to the carnivore diet.

Slow Cooker Pulled Pork

What's inside:

Butter (1 tbsp.)
Celtic sea salt
Chicken broth (.5 c.)
Pork shoulder roast (4 lbs.)

How to make:

1. To start this recipe, bring out your slow cooker and get it set up. When it is ready, add the pork roast to the bottom.
2. Add in the broth, salt, and butter all around the pork roast and then cover up the slow cooker.
3. Turn this onto a low setting and let it cook. After seven hours, you can turn off the slow cooker.
4. Take the pork roast out of the slow cooker and allow it to cool down for a few minutes.
5. Use either your hands or a fork to shred the pork and then place the shredded pork back into the slow cooker.

6. Stir the shredded meat around to make sure that it is covered up in the juices and then serve warm.

Chicken and Pork Rind

What's inside:

Salt
Butter (2 tbsp.)
Eggs (2)
Pork rinds, ground (1 bag)
Chicken breasts (300 g.)

How to make:

1. Take out the chicken and use salt to season it. In another bowl, crack and whip the eggs to make your batter.
2. Take out a plate and thinly spread the pork crumbs out on it.
3. When you are ready, take the prepared chicken and dip it first into the bowl with the beaten egg. Shake it a bit to remove the extra liquid, then dip the chicken into the bread crumbs.
4. You can choose to either bake or pan-sear the chicken. After you have done that, spread out the butter and then bake some more.
5. Once the chicken has turned golden brown in color, the meal is ready for you to serve.

Bacon and Shredded Chicken

What's inside:

Slow cooked chicken breast (1)
Pepper (1 tbsp.)
Salt (1 tbsp.)
Butter (2 tbsp.)
Chopped bacon slices (1)

How to make:

1. To start, take out the slow cooker and get it set up. Add the chicken inside and let it cook on a low setting.
2. After five hours, take the chicken out of the slow cooker and use your hands or a fork to shred it up.
3. Take out a skillet and add some butter. When the butter is melted, pan fry the bacon.
4. Once the bacon starts to produce some fats, add in the shredded chicken to this and cook for a bit.
5. After five minutes, season with pepper and salt that you want and then serve the dish.

Southern Steak

What's inside:

Salt (1 tsp.)
Chopped sirloin steaks (2 lbs.)
Water (3 c.)
Beef broth (.5 c.)
Butter (5 tbsp.)
Pepper (1 tsp.)

How to make:

1. Take out the pieces of steak and season it with some pepper and salt to start.
2. When that is done, take out a big pan or a skillet and add the butter. Once the butter has some time to melt, you can add in the steaks and let them cook for a bit.
3. Cook the steaks until they start to brown a bit on each side. Then take the steaks out of the pan and set them inside your prepared slow cooker.
4. Inside the skillet, add in the three cups of water along with the broth. Reduce your heat to medium high and bring these liquids to a boil.
5. Once this is boiling, add the mixture to the slow cooker. Cover up the cooker and set it to a low setting.
6. After eight hours, you can turn off the slow cooker and take the meat out to serve.

Roasted Cream Chicken and Bone Broth

What's inside:

Heavy whipping cream (2 c.)
Salt
Whole chicken (4 lbs.)
Ghee (3 tbsp.)

How to make:

1. Take the chicken out of the fridge and let it set on the counter for some time. Give it about an hour to warm up.
2. After this time, turn the oven on and give it time to heat up to 325 degrees. While the oven is heating up, you can take the whipping cream out of the fridge and let it heat up a little bit.
3. Now take out the chicken and pat it dry with some paper towels. Season the chicken generously with some salt, both on the inside and the outside.
4. Bring out your Dutch oven and let it start to heat up on the stove. Add in a bit of ghee to this before adding in the chicken.
5. Brown the chicken for about five minutes on each side in the Dutch oven. When the chicken is done with the browning process, add in the whipping cream to the Dutch oven as well.
6. Place the lid onto the Dutch oven and add it to the oven to bake. After 60 minutes, you can check to see if the chicken has reached the right temperature.
7. Let the chicken rest for a few minutes after you take it out of the oven and then carve. Serve the chicken with some cream and then serve.

Pan Roasted Duck Breast

What's inside:

Salt
Deboned duck breast

How to make:

1. Take the duck breast out of the fridge and give it time to warm up to room temperature before you cook it. This can take about an hour.
2. Score the fat and skin with a sharp knife in a criss-cross pattern, making sure that you don't cut into the meat too much. Season with salt on all sides.
3. Turn on the oven and let it heat up to 350 degrees. Get an oven safe skillet nice and hot. Once the skillet is hot, you can add the duck breast in, making sure that the skin side is down.
4. Cook this for ten minutes or so. Turn down the heat a bit if you notice that the skin is getting too hot.
5. After you sear all of the sides, go and put the skin side down before transferring it to the oven for a bit.
6. After another five to six minutes, the duck should be cooked all the way through at least 165 degrees.
7. After the duck reaches this temperature, take it out of the oven and let it cool down before slicing and serving.

Pork Tenderloin on the Stove

What's inside:

Salt
Pork tenderloin

How to make:

1. Turn on the oven and give it time to heat up to 350 degrees. Use a boning knife to help you to remove any silver skin on the tenderloin. You can then cut the pork into medallions or leave it as a whole.
2. Use salt to season the pork on all sides. Take out a skillet that is safe for the oven and let it get hot on the stove. Add in a bit of ghee or bacon fat.
3. Once the bacon fat or ghee is warmed up, cook the pork inside. Cook this on all sides for about a minute.
4. After this time, you can move the pork over to the oven and let it cook. This will take about ten minutes to complete.
5. Let the pork rest for ten minutes or so and then slice up before serving.

Roasted Turkey

What's inside:

Softened ghee (6 tbsp.)
Salt
Turkey, with the neck and giblets removed (12 lbs.)

How to make:

1. Take the turkey out of the fridge and let it set on the counter for 30 minutes. Then take some time to break it down.
2. Turn on the oven and give it some time to heat up to 450 degrees. Move the rack to the lower third of your oven to prepare it.
3. Pat the turkey dry and then pull the skin away from the meat a bit, but don't pull it all the way off.
4. Slid parts of the butter or ghee between the meat and the skin as you can, and then lay the skin back over. Season the whole turkey with some salt.
5. Add the turkey parts to your roasting pan and place into the oven to bake. After 25 minutes, turn the heat of the oven down to 325 degrees. Take a moment to baste the turkey with all of its juices.
6. After another 30 minutes, check to see the temperature of the turkey. You want the breast to be at least 145 degrees and the thighs and legs to be 165 degrees.
7. Once the turkey has reached the right temperature, take it out of the oven and give it ten to fifteen minutes to cool down. Serve warm.

Slow Cooker Beef Tongue

What's inside:

Water or bone broth (1 quart)
Salt
Rinsed beef tongue (4 lbs.)

How to make:

1. Rinse the beef tongue off. Lay it out flat and then season with some salt before adding to your prepared slow cooker.
2. Make sure to add enough of the water or the broth to cover the tongue up, and then place the lid on top of the slow cooker.
3. Turn the slow cooker on to the low setting to cook. After ten hours, turn the slow cooker off. Carefully remove the hot tongue and pull the skin off gently. At this point, it should come off pretty easily.
4. Now, slice up the beef and sear it in a skillet with some hot butter. You can also choose to shred the beef with the help of two forks.
5. Season with more salt if needed before serving. Keep the leftover liquid to use as a stock.

Oyster Cream Panfry

What's inside:

Salt
Heavy cream (.5 c.)
Bone broth (.25 c.)
Ghee or butter (1 tsp.)
Shucked fresh oysters (12)

How to make:

1. To start this recipe, add the oysters to a small pan. Heat up some of the butter or ghee on medium heat and start cooking.
2. Pour the broth on top. When it begins to simmer and froth, gently stir the oysters until their edges begin to turn.
3. After this time, add in the cream and bring it to a simmer. Season the whole thing with some salt and take the pan off the heat.
4. Allow your oysters to sit in the sauce for a few minutes to warm up and soak in the sauce. Transfer this dish to some bowls and then serve.

Steamed Clams or Mussels

What's inside:

Mussels (1 lb. per person)
Bone broth (.5 c.)
Ghee (2 tbsp.)

How to make:

1. Take out a big pot that has a lid. Add in the ghee or some butter and let it melt on medium heat.
2. After the butter has some time to melt, add in the bone broth and the mussels to the pot. Add the lid to the top.
3. Turn the heat of the stove to high setting and cook these for a bit. After three minutes, shake the pot a bit, making sure that the lid is still on, and rotate the mussels.
4. Let these cook for a bit longer. After another 5 minutes, you can take the pot off the heat. Take the mussels out of the pot and place into a serving bowl.
5. Ladle the broth over the mussels, but make sure to leave the sediment that is there at the bottom of the pot and enjoy.

Chicken Livers Wrapped with Bacon

What's inside:

Ghee or butter (3 oz.)
Bacon, cut in half (.5 lbs.)
Chicken livers (1 lb.)

How to make:

1. Take the butter and place it into a pan to heat up and become melted.
2. Once the butter or ghee is melted, you can add in the chicken livers and let it brown on both sides before taking them out of the heat.
3. Take a half strip of bacon and wrap it around each of the pieces of chicken livers. Secure the bacon in place with some toothpicks.
4. Add these back into the skillet and pan fry the livers and the bacon until the bacon has become nice and crisp.
5. Once this happens, take the chicken livers and bacon out of the skillet, take the toothpicks out of the meats, and then serve this warm.

Slow Cooker Chicken Gizzards

What's inside:

Pepper
Salt
Beef broth (8 c.)
Chicken hearts (1 bag)
Chicken gizzards (1 bag)

How to make:

1. To start this recipe, you can take the chicken parts and rinse them with some water.
2. Set up the slow cooker and then add the gizzards inside first. Then add in the chicken hearts and add the pepper and salt.
3. Cover the gizzards and the heart with some of the beef broth and then add the lid onto the slow cooker.
4. Put the slow cooker on a heat setting that is low. After eight hours, the chicken parts will be done and you can serve warm.

Conclusion

Thank you for making it through to the end of *Carnivore Diet*. Let's hope it was informative and able to provide you with all of the tools you need to achieve your goals whatever they may be.

The next step is to get started on the carnivore diet and see if it is the right choice for you. There are a lot of different diet plans out there and many times, they end up contradicting each other and confusing the person who is trying to go on them. Some of them may work but are too hard to maintain for a long period of time, and others may be easier, but they just don't work at all. This can leave the dieter feeling like a failure, and they wonder if they can ever lose the weight and feel good again.

The carnivore diet is going to be a bit different than this. Instead of making up a bunch of complicated rules that are hard to follow, the carnivore diet is going to instead focus on keeping things simple and taking us back to our roots. On this diet plan, you will focus on just eating animal products. This means lots of meat, including fish, eggs, butter, and some aged cheese. Outside of that, the other foods need to be avoided.

Those who follow this kind of diet plan are going to see some great results. You will find that there are a few weeks of transitioning away from the traditional foods that you like to enjoy, including the carbs, sugars, and even produce. But once the body adjusts and you see some of the great meals that you are able to enjoy on this plan, you will be wondering why you didn't try this out before!

This guidebook took some time to talk about the carnivore diet and all of the steps that you can take to see some results with it. There is so much to love when it comes to this diet plan, and if you are able to get on it and maintain it, you are sure to see the results.

Inside this guidebook, we have given you the steps that you need to see some great results. We talked about the basics of this diet plan, the foods that you are allowed to consume, the way that exercise can fit into the plan, and so much more. You even get the benefit of seeing some delicious meals and a full meal plan that can make this diet plan the best option for you.

If you are tired of dieting and getting confused by all of the rules and recommendations that come with other diet plans, and you want a plan that actually works and is simple to keep up with, the carnivore diet might be the best one for you.

Finally, if you found this book useful in any way, a review on Amazon is always appreciated!

www.ingramcontent.com/pod-product-compliance
Lightning Source LLC
Chambersburg PA
CBHW020309290526
45784CB00003B/1425